W9-CEJ-617

THE HEARING LOSS HANDBOOK

THE HEARING LOSS HANDBOOK

David M. Vernick, M.D.
Constance Grzelka
and the Editors of
Consumer Reports Books

CONSUMER REPORTS BOOKS
A Division of Consumers Union
Yonkers, New York

Published by Consumers Union of United States, Inc.,
Yonkers, New York 10703.

Library of Congress Cataloging-in-Publication Data

Vernick, David M.
The hearing loss handbook / David M. Vernick, Constance Grzelka,
and the Editors of Consumer Reports Books.
p. cm.
Includes bibliographical references and index.
ISBN-0-89043-576-6
1. Deafness—Popular works. 2. Hearing disorders—Popular works.
3. Consumer education. I. Grzelka, Constance. II. Consumer
Reports Books. III. Title.
RF291.35.V47 1993
617.8—dc20 93-2607
CIP

Drawings by Phyllis Wood. Drawings on pages 17 and 79 by Harriet Greenfield.
Design by GDS/Jeffrey L. Ward
First printing, October 1993
Manufactured in the United States of America

This book was printed on recycled paper

The Hearing Loss Handbook is a Consumer Reports Book published by Consumers Union, the nonprofit organization that publishes *Consumer Reports*, the monthly magazine of test reports, product Ratings, and buying guidance. Established in 1936, Consumers Union is chartered under the Not-for-Profit Corporation Law of the State of New York.

The purposes of Consumers Union, as stated in its charter, are to provide consumers with information and counsel on consumer goods and services, to give information on all matters relating to the expenditure of the family income, and to initiate and to cooperate with individual and group efforts seeking to create and maintain decent living standards.

Consumers Union derives its income solely from the sale of *Consumer Reports* and other publications. In addition, expenses of occasional public service efforts may be met, in part, by nonrestrictive, noncommercial contributions, grants, and fees. Consumers Union accepts no advertising or product samples and is not beholden in any way to any commercial interest. Its Ratings and reports are solely for the use of the readers of its publications. Neither the Ratings, nor the reports, nor any Consumers Union publications, including this book, may be used in advertising or for any commercial purpose. Consumers Union will take all steps open to it to prevent such uses of its material, its name, or the name of *Consumer Reports*.

To my loving wife, Mary,
and my super kids, Gregory and Christopher,
for their inspiration and support.

—David M. Vernick, M.D.

To my mother, Nellie Grzelka,
and to the loving memory
of my father, Chester J. Grzelka.

—Constance Grzelka

The ideas and suggestions contained in this book are not intended to replace the services of a physician. All matters regarding health require medical supervision, and the reader should consult a physician or other health professional before adopting the procedures outlined in *The Hearing Loss Handbook*. Any use of the procedures discussed in this book is at the reader's discretion, and neither the authors nor the publisher assumes any responsibility or liability for any such use.

The reader should also consult a physician or health professional before purchasing or using any hearing device described or evaluated in this book. Neither the authors nor the publisher endorses any particular hearing aid, listening device, or product discussed or listed in these pages.

CONTENTS

ACKNOWLEDGMENTS

The authors would like to thank the hearing health-care professionals and educators who shared their knowledge and offered guidance that was instrumental in creating various sections of this book. Their dedication to the men, women, and children with hearing loss is impressive and inspiring.

Special thanks go to Terri Loewenthal, M.S., CCC-A, audiologist at the Joint Center for Otolaryngology, Boston; Dennis Gjerdingen, President of Clarke School for the Deaf in Northampton, Massachusetts, and his staff; Steven C. White, Ph.D., Director of the Healthcare Financing Division, American Speech-Language-Hearing Association, Rockville, Maryland; Elizabeth Ewell, National Center on Employment of the Deaf, Rochester, New York; William J. Mahon, Hearing Industries Association, Washington, D.C.; and Kenneth W. Berger, Ph.D., Professor Emeritus of Audiology, Kent State University, Kent, Ohio.

A special thank-you to Estrellita Karsh for her insightful review and suggestions. A note of appreciation also is due to Linda Piccirilli, R.N., for her technical assistance and support. Finally, thanks to Julie Henderson for her editorial guidance and help in the production of this book.

Introduction

Hearing loss affects millions of Americans. As life expectancy in this country continues to increase, the number of hearing-impaired people is expected to rise as well. It has been estimated that by the middle of the twenty-first century, more than 36 million people will have some form of hearing loss.

Hearing loss isn't a life-threatening disorder. Instead, it cuts off the hard-of-hearing or deaf person from other people, leaving them socially bereft. The legendary Helen Keller, who was blind as well as deaf, came to the conclusion that "to be deaf is a greater affliction than to be blind. . . . To be cut off from hearing is to be isolated indeed."

For many centuries, there was a great deal of ignorance about hearing loss and much scorn was directed toward the deaf. Despite the many medical, surgical, and technological advances that have since been discovered to treat hearing loss, there still remains today a great reluctance on the part of many to acknowledge a hearing problem—even when help is available. Fortunately, a growing awareness of the importance of good hearing is finally bringing the issue of hearing loss into the open.

Publicity also helps. When former president Ronald Reagan first appeared before the nation wearing a hearing aid in 1983, public acceptance of hearing devices increased dramatically. Many people who formerly were reluctant to wear a hearing aid now felt more comfortable about seeking help for their hearing impairment.

A major sign of government support for identifying and preventing problems that can lead to hearing loss was the creation in 1988 of the National Institute on Deafness and Other Communication Disorders.

This newest member of the National Institutes of Health (NIH) conducts and supports research on hearing as well as on balance, speech, and language. With the inception of many new programs, it is hoped that hearing and other communication disorders will receive the attention—and funding—necessary to help solve some of the problems related to hearing loss.

WHO NEEDS THIS BOOK

Hearing loss is widespread and occurs most commonly in the elderly, who constitute a rapidly growing segment of the population. But many teenagers and young adults are beginning to show signs of hearing loss as a result of exposure to noise-related recreational activities.

When a child suffers from hearing loss, the situation becomes even more critical. The amount and type of special training necessary to develop communication skills will depend on whether the child was born deaf or became hearing-impaired after beginning to learn language.

To lose one's hearing is physically and emotionally devastating. Too many people prefer not to think about it; others would like more information but don't know where to start. This book can answer many of the basic questions you may have about your hearing, the professionals who provide hearing health care and other related services, and the interventions now available for treating hearing loss.

HOW TO USE THIS BOOK

The Hearing Loss Handbook is not necessarily intended to be read from cover to cover. You may want to read certain chapters to obtain a general understanding of how the human hearing mechanism works or to find out what measures you can take to prevent hearing loss. If you have been experiencing a particular problem or are seeking more information on a range of topics—from hearing aids to dizziness—you may want to turn to that specific subject area and learn more about it.

The amazing story of how we hear is a good place to begin in understanding how hearing loss can occur in that complex and highly sensitive organ—the human ear. The body's crucial system of balance, also located in the ear, can be affected as well. Chapter 1 discusses the structure and workings of the human auditory system.

Hearing loss has many causes. Some may affect only the outer ear, whereas others may occur inside the middle ear or deep within the inner ear. As you will learn in chapter 2, there are some problems that may be self-limiting and clear up on their own; others, however, call for immediate medical attention.

The discovery of a hearing loss comes as a shock to everyone—especially the parents of an infant who gradually realize that their baby isn't responding to sound. Chapter 3 provides an idea of what such a diagnosis means for adults as well as for children, and it also explains how hearing is tested.

Hearing aids have long had a negative image. Their poor reputation was mainly based on stories of people who bought shoddy or badly fitted instruments. Chapter 4 goes into detail about the different types, styles, and capabilities of the various hearing devices on the market today. This chapter also includes practical advice on how to deal with hearing aid dispensers.

When medical treatment or a hearing aid can't resolve a hearing problem, then surgery may be called for. An important new treatment option for deafness is a cochlear implant, an operation in which an electronic device is surgically implanted in the inner ear. Chapter 5 describes how cochlear implants work, who is best suited for them, and what you can expect if you choose this procedure.

Other hearing aids, known as assistive listening devices, help make communication easier. These devices are discussed in chapter 6, including descriptions of the most popular ones on the market, their advantages and drawbacks, and how to use them.

Preventing hearing loss that is caused by exposure to noise is covered in chapter 7. The risks from certain illnesses, infections, drugs, chemicals, and abrupt pressure changes are also described.

As mentioned previously, your ears also contain delicate and highly complex organs affecting balance. When infection, injury, or some other problem disturbs your vestibular (balancing) system, then you may experience a host of symptoms, including dizziness and vertigo. Balance disorders as well as other problems of the ear, such as the constant noise of tinnitus and the disturbing symptoms of Ménière's disease—and what to do about them—are also discussed in chapter 8.

Living with hearing loss is a learned behavior. Adults who have a hearing problem can use the many coping skills and strategies provided in chapter 9. For the parents of a deaf child, there are suggestions on finding the right professionals, dealing with the local school system, and the different philosophies of hearing education in use today among the hearing-impaired. By knowing all of the options that are available, parents have the opportunity to make an informed decision on how to best educate a child with hearing loss.

Chapter 10 discusses how to choose hearing care. It tells you what to look for in the different professionals who provide hearing-care services and how you can find the right people for your needs. The economics of health care are also included in this chapter, including what you can expect from insurance companies in terms of reimbursement for costs. If you need a hearing aid or other listening device but don't have insurance coverage or can't affort to pay for it, there is a section here on where you might look for assistance.

The appendixes provide a wide range of information. First, you will find the results of the latest evaluations of hearing aids by the Department of Veterans Affairs. Also included are a report by the technical staff of *Consumer Reports* magazine on various popular types of assistive listening devices and a listing of self-help groups and other sources of information.

If knowledge is power, then the purpose of this book is to provide hearing-impaired and deaf individuals with the most up-to-date and accurate information to help them help themselves. The world may be made for the normal-hearing person, but new technology and a wide range of interventions can help make that world accessible to all people with hearing problems.

1

Sound and the Structure of the Ear

Many people complain about the size and shape of their ears. But it's what is inside that really counts.

Your ears are highly sensitive and complex organs that govern the body's sense of hearing as well as balance. As a sensory organ, a properly working ear will enable you to communicate with the external world, to interpret sounds that make their way to your brain, and to experience the entire aural array that surrounds you daily.

Various parts, systems, and connections exist within the ear that allow sound to eventually reach the brain. All are essential components of hearing. But before discussing this amazing auditory apparatus, it's necessary to understand the origin and significance of sound.

SOUND

Sound is a form of energy that passes through the ear and registers in the brain as something that is heard. Essentially, sound is simply vibrating air molecules. These quivering tiny particles of air can be produced by the characteristic whine of the rapidly beating wings of a mosquito, by the twang of guitar strings, or by the roar of baseball fans in an enclosed stadium. Depending on the situation, the sound in your ear and brain may be pleasurable, frightening, or just plain annoying.

Characteristics of Sound

Sound is measured by its frequency and force, or loudness.

Frequency. What you hear and how well you hear it depends on the frequency and intensity of sound. Ever wonder why lightning flashes occur first during a storm, followed later by a clap of thunder? It's because sound travels at the speed of about 1,100 feet per second (about a fifth of a mile), while light moves much more rapidly, at 186,282 miles per second. But although sound is slower, its power can be formidable. The ear is capable of hearing a wide range of sounds—from the barely audible to those that are so loud they produce pain and damage hearing.

You can feel some sounds as well as hear them. For example, it's possible to feel a vibration in your chest when the speakers in some stereo systems are operating at a certain frequency. Similarly, the low rumble of New York subway trains that are several levels underground can be felt on the first floor of some buildings in the city.

The frequency of a sound wave is measured by means of a unit called *hertz*. If a sound travels slowly, it has a low number of cycles per second, or hertz, as well as a low tone. A fast-moving sound has a higher frequency and produces a higher tone.

The human ear is capable of responding to a wide range of frequencies, from lows of about 20 hertz to highs of about 20,000 hertz. The speaking frequency for most people falls into the 500-to-2,000-hertz range. The ear is most sensitive to sounds that are 1,000 to 4,000 hertz.

Because the ear is sensitive to different sounds at different levels of intensities, certain tones can cause more damage to the ear than others. The most sensitive area is at 4,000 hertz. If you were exposed to a collection of all tones played at once—this is known as *white noise*—the damage to your hearing would first occur at 4,000 hertz. Since most loud noises are similar to white noise, you can see how hearing loss can easily happen.

Hearing is at its keenest during childhood, when it is possible to hear frequencies as low as 16 hertz and, in some cases, as high as 40,000 hertz. But the ability to hear so acutely begins to drop after about age 10.

Loudness. The relative power or force contained in a sound—its loudness—is measured in *decibels*. The term *decibel* (dB) is derived from both a number and a person: "Deci" indicates one-tenth of a

Extremes of Sound Frequency: Infrasound and Ultrasound

Sounds that vibrate at frequencies below the lowest level of human hearing, at 20 hertz, are called *infrasound*. The primary natural source of infrasonic sound waves is earthquakes.

High-frequency sound waves that range above the highest level of human hearing, at 20,000 hertz, are known as *ultrasound*. Bats, birds, cats, dogs, dolphins, and whales are among the animals that communicate via ultrasonic waves.

An early practical application of ultrasound was sonar, first used during World War II for the detection of underwater objects such as submarines. Sonar sends high-pitched sound waves toward a target and has them reflect back to the sender, a process called echolocation.

Medical scientists have also discovered many uses for ultrasound in both diagnosing and treating a variety of ailments. Ultrasound imaging is now used to detect heart abnormalities, blood clots, aneurysms, detached retinas, kidney stones, and tumors. Doctors may order ultrasound imaging for pregnant women in order to determine whether the fetus is growing normally. No evidence has been found to show that any damage results to the developing fetus from ultrasound testing, even if multiple ultrasound tests are performed. Ultrasound is also used in the treatment of certain forms of glaucoma and for the relief of pain and stiffness in joints and muscles.

number, and "bel" is a tribute to Alexander Graham Bell, inventor of the telephone. Decibels cannot be compared to units of measurement, like inches or pounds. They are more like the f-stops that are found on a camera lens.

The decibel scale is a logarithmic progression much like the Richter scale is for seismic activity. It is multiplied by 10 for every tenfold increase in sound intensity. Therefore, a sound that is 10 dB is 10 times louder than something that measures 0 dB. Adding 20 dB makes a sound 100 times as loud, whereas an increase of 30 dB makes it 1,000

WHAT'S THAT NOISE?

Decibel Level	Sound
0	Faintest sound heard by human ear
30	Whisper, quiet library
60	Normal conversation, sewing machine, typewriter
90	Lawn mower, shop tools, truck traffic
100	Chain saw, pneumatic drill, snowmobile
115	Sandblasting, loud rock concert, automobile horn
140	Gun muzzle blast, jet engine

Source: American Academy of Otolaryngology—Head and Neck Surgery, Inc.

times louder. An additional 50 dB would increase the intensity 100,000 times.

The faintest sound the human ear can hear is 0 dB, the lowest level on the decibel scale, and basically the threshold of hearing. The loudest sound—the roar of a rocket lifting off from its launch pad—registers at more than 180 dB.

A device called a sound level meter is used to physically measure the pressure of sounds in the environment. The meter takes an average reading of the amount of sound over a period of time (e.g., one second). Then, using a special scale, the meter makes the closest approximation to the hearing level of the human ear.

Three different scales are used in sound level meters to analyze the sound pressure of various frequency bands: the A-, B-, and C-scales. Because the frequency response of the A-scale comes the closest to what the human ear hears as sound, it is used for most sound analysis.

Sound level meters vary in their sensitivity and sophistication. A variety of these instruments are available, ranging from the fairly complex and expensive to simpler devices found in electronics stores.

Pathways of Sound

However soft or loud, sound travels to the ear by means of sound waves. The outer ear helps to funnel the sound waves through the ear canal to the eardrum, which vibrates when the sound strikes it. The vibrating eardrum then transmits the waves of sound to bones in the middle ear.

It is at the end of this stage of sound transmission that sound waves change from vibrations in the air (outer ear) and in bone (middle ear) to vibrations in the fluid-filled environment of the inner ear. Specialized sensory cells in the inner ear immediately convert the incoming fluid waves into electrical impulses, or nerve signals, for transmission to the brain.

Sound transmission through the pathways of the ear meets some resistance, however. The waves bounce off many surfaces during their transit, and much of their energy may be lost because of a phenomenon called reflection. Fortunately, the structures of the middle ear intensify sound and help make up for the lost sound energy.

It also takes much more energy to transmit sound waves through the fluid of the inner ear than it does to move them through air or bone. This becomes clearer if you consider that walking through water takes much more energy than walking at the same pace along the edge of the sea. And so it is with sound that enters the inner ear: More energy is needed to travel through its fluid interior.

THE STRUCTURE OF THE EAR

As we have seen, the human ear has three distinct parts—the outer ear, the middle ear, and the inner ear. All of these components receive, amplify, and transmit tones to the brain. These tones are then recognized as sounds.

The Outer Ear

The external ear begins with the *auricle*, the shell-like flap of cartilage and skin located on either side of the head. The auricle helps to

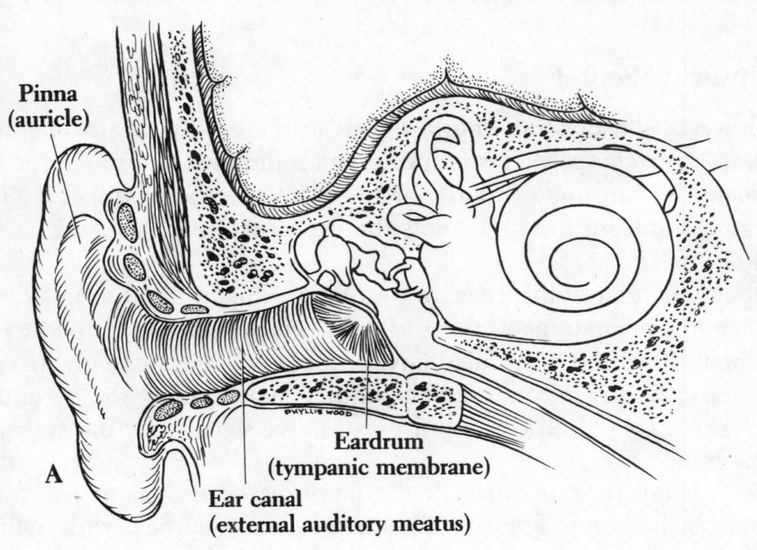

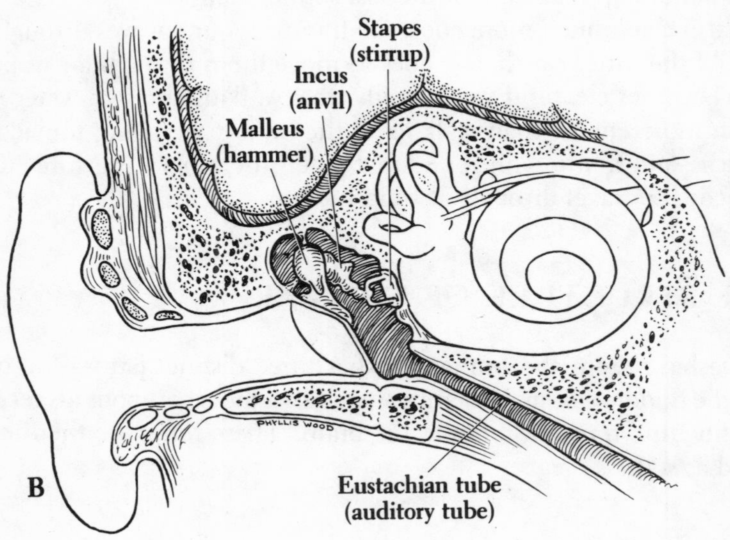

The outer ear (A) and the middle ear (B)

gather and direct sound waves into the ear canal, the inch-long passageway that leads to the eardrum.

The skin lining the outer part of the ear canal contains hair follicles, sebaceous glands, and glands that produce *cerumen*, or earwax. The tiny hairs of the ear act like a filter, keeping out dust and dirt just as the hairs in the nose help prevent incoming debris from traveling to the lungs. The skin in the ear canal goes through the same processes as other body skin; dead skin cells rise to the top layer and slough off so that new ones can take their place. As skin cells are shed, they mix with earwax and work their way out of the ear canal.

The ear secretes cerumen for several reasons: to clean the ear canal, to keep the flow of dirt and debris moving to the outside and away from the inner portion of the ear canal, and to lubricate the delicate skin.

At the end of the ear canal lies the eardrum, or tympanic membrane. It forms a tight seal between the outer ear and the adjoining area—the middle ear. The eardrum measures about a half-inch in diameter, has the thickness of a strand of hair, and is normally pearly gray in color. Under examination, the tympanic membrane gives the impression of looking through wax paper. Under the light of an examining instrument called an otoscope, it's possible to see shadows of what's on the other side. While examining the eardrum, the physician also observes its appearance, position, ability to vibrate, and color. When the eardrum is red, for example, it indicates inflammation. A yellow-tinged eardrum points to fluid behind the membrane.

The eardrum tends to get more opaque with age, making it more difficult to see through it. Thickening of the eardrum doesn't necessarily only occur with age; repeated infections can lead to scarring that also causes it to thicken.

Three layers of tissue make up the tympanic membrane. Skin forms the dry outer layer that faces the ear canal. The middle layer is composed of connective tissue such as fibrin and collagen, which makes it taut and stiff. The inside layer, facing the middle ear, has a mucosal lining like the interior of the mouth and nose.

It's common to think of the eardrum as a flat, round disk—but its shape is really concave. The center points inward, somewhat like the cone-shaped speaker of a stereo system.

The Middle Ear

The middle ear is an air-filled chamber about as large as a shelled peanut. It contains three tiny bones collectively known as the *ossicles*.

The ossicles consist of the malleus, incus, and stapes (popularly known as the hammer, anvil, and stirrup because of their different shapes).

This trio of bones links up to form a bridge across the middle-ear cavity. The outer end of the malleus is attached to the eardrum. Its opposite side fits into the adjoining bone, the incus. The incus in turn connects with the stapes. Tiny ligaments attached to the walls and roof of the middle ear help to keep these bones in place. The stapes sits directly at the entrance to the inner ear and actually fills the opening—called the *oval window*—into the inner ear. The stapes is held in place by a circular ligament that attaches to the area around the window.

Any sound that enters the ear through the ear canal passes through

The Evolution of Hearing

Human hearing, with its ability to discriminate and make sense of a wide range of sound frequencies, is a highly complex activity.

Not all animals hear the way we do, but instead have a variety of specialized sensors that register changes in the outer environment or in the body itself. Many of their sense structures aren't recognizable as ears—at least not as we know them—but these structures do receive sound waves and allow the animal to respond to the stimulus in accordance with its nature.

One of the earliest forms of sound receptors is found in fish—a string of fluid-filled sensors called lateral line organs, which detect vibration and pressure changes in the water. As water-dwelling creatures moved to dry land, they had to develop sound receptors that were more responsive to sound waves traveling through the air. They also needed a more advanced system of maintaining body balance than the simple set of liquid-filled sacs of the ancient fish.

Insects have developed a sense of hearing that relies on simple but specialized auditory structures. Hearing organs, for example, appear on the legs of katydids and on the abdomens of grasshoppers. Mosquitoes have an organ at the base of each antenna that contains sensory units called scolophores, and these apparently serve as sound receptors.

Snakes don't have an outer or middle ear but have a long bone called a columnella, which leads to the inner ear. Although snakes aren't very sensitive to sounds in the air, they have a keen sense of sounds that vibrate through the ground.

Birds are similar to reptiles in that they have a single long bone that transmits vibrations to the inner ear. However, birds actually have a longer and more sensitive cochlea that is able to distinguish the pitch of sounds in frequencies well above the limit discerned by humans.

Mammals, including dogs, cats, horses, and deer, have the three distinct parts of the ear—outer ear, middle ear, and inner ear. The coiled cochlea of the inner ear, with its sensitive hair cells, allows them to determine such characteristics of sound as pitch. Many of these animals can detect sounds in frequency ranges much higher than the human ear is capable of hearing. Cats have a hearing range of 25,000 hertz, whereas dogs can hear sounds up to 35,000. (The human ear can hear sounds up to 20,000 hertz.)

Among the more mystifying hearing organs in the animal world are those of bats and dolphins. These mammals have a highly developed auditory sense and are renowned for their power of echolocation, a form of acoustic radar. In echolocation, the animal transmits a series of high-pitched sounds, then listens for the echoes that are reflected back. This ability enables an animal to either avoid the objects that produce the echoes, or, in the case of bats, to precisely pinpoint the position of their prey—small insects—and catch them on the wing.

the eardrum and is converted from sound energy in the air to mechanical energy when it reaches the middle ear. Given the size of the eardrum (which is some 20 times larger than the oval window) and the amplification power of the ossicles, this incoming sound is highly concentrated by the time it vibrates through the stapes and is transmitted into the oval window.

The middle ear can amplify sound, but it also can decrease or muffle sound heading toward the inner ear. This dampening effect, which is thought to be a protective function, is accomplished by two small muscles. The first of these muscles, called the *tensor tympani*, attaches to the first bone of hearing, the malleus. The other muscle—the *stapedius*—is attached to the stapes.

The tensing action of these muscles—the so-called acoustic reflex—reduces the efficiency of sound being transmitted through the ossicles. Although the tensor tympani and the stapedius appear to protect the hearing mechanism to some degree, they are not effective against impact noise such as a gun being fired close to the ear.

The middle ear has a mucosal lining and contains the opening to the *eustachian tube*, a narrow vent that links the middle ear and the throat. Air enters or leaves the tube when you swallow and yawn, ventilating the middle ear and equalizing the pressure on the interior with the atmospheric pressure on the other side of the eardrum. When there is a pressure difference between the middle ear and the outside world, as can occur when a plane descends to land, pressure and pain (aerotitis) can result.

At the top of the middle-ear cavity is a small space that opens into the mastoid, a bony mucosal-lined area that is actually part of the skull. The mastoid area is filled with small spikes of bone. Its function remains unknown.

The Inner Ear

The inner ear is the most complex part of the organ of hearing. Although the inner ear occupies a small space—about the size of a cherry—it contains extremely elaborate structures that affect both hearing and balance. Its construction is so intricate and involved that it has been called a "labyrinth inside a labyrinth."

The first major component of the inner ear is the *cochlea*, a snail-shaped structure that spirals around itself for two and a half turns. The mechanism inside the cochlea is central to the hearing process, for this is where sound energy that has passed through the middle ear is transformed into nerve signals that the brain perceives as sound.

The other component within the chamber of the inner ear is the *labyrinth*, with its curlicue course of loops, the *semicircular canals*. This structure and its contents literally keeps us from going in circles because it governs the body's sense of balance and equilibrium.

Although the cochlea and the labyrinth have different responsibilities, they are nevertheless connected. When one of these inner-ear components isn't working properly, it can affect the function of the other.

These delicate and sensitive structures are among the body's best-protected organs. The inner ear lies deep inside the temporal bone of the skull, surrounded by some of the densest bone in the body. Let's examine how these two vital parts work.

THE COCHLEA

The cochlea is composed of a bony outer cavity and a membranous inside cavity. Each of these areas has a particular fluid environment. The bony space of the inner ear floats in a fluid called *perilymph*, a watery substance similar in composition to spinal fluid and the aqueous humor in the front of the eyeball. Another fluid—also with the consistency of water—is called *endolymph* and is found inside the membranous cavity of the cochlea.

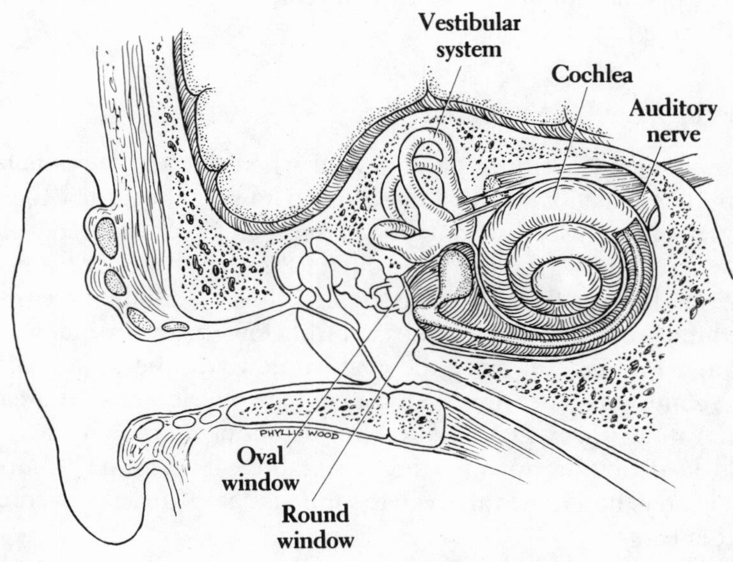

The inner ear

The endolymph exists in an essentially self-contained system. The perilymph surrounds the membranes that contain the endolymph. To clarify this arrangement of fluids inside the inner ear, think of a fluid-filled balloon inside a bucket of fluid that has a similar consistency but a different composition. The bucket water is the perilymph and the water inside the balloon is the endolymph.

Both of these fluids contain electrolytes—substances that can conduct an electrical charge. Endolymph has a high concentration of potassium, while perilymph has a high sodium content. This sets up an electrical field. When a wave of sound stimulates the inner ear hair cells, chemicals are released that alter the electrical field and thus excite the appropriate sensory nerve cells, resulting in the sensation of sound.

Normally, the perilymph and endolymph don't mix. When the fluids do combine or leak, this can indicate a disease or a disorder of the inner ear. For instance, people who produce too much endolymph may develop a condition called Ménière's disease (see chapter 8). Using the example of the balloon in the bucket, imagine that the fluid-filled balloon keeps swelling until it ruptures, which is what happens in Ménière's disease. When the two different fluids mix, the combination essentially short-circuits the system and results in an attack of dizziness and hearing impairment.

How the Cochlea Functions

Sound energy gets into the inner ear when the tiny stapes bone in the middle ear vibrates, or "raps," on a membrane called the oval window—in a sense, the front door of the cochlea. Once inside, sound becomes a fluid wave: Its energy circles through this coiled tube and then spirals back through to its final pathway—another membrane called the "round window" that sits just below the oval window.

Sound waves never strike the oval window and the round window at the same time, because such a simultaneous action would cancel out the fluid waves that produce the incoming sound. In fact, you would hear nothing in this kind of situation. The round window is considered to be a relief valve where sound is dampened as it eventually exits the ear.

The fluid sound wave that surges into the cochlea sweeps past a layer of cells on the basilar membrane. This is a tablelike structure that supports the sensory hair cells lining the cochlea. The sound wave causes a vibration along the basilar membrane. Different regions along

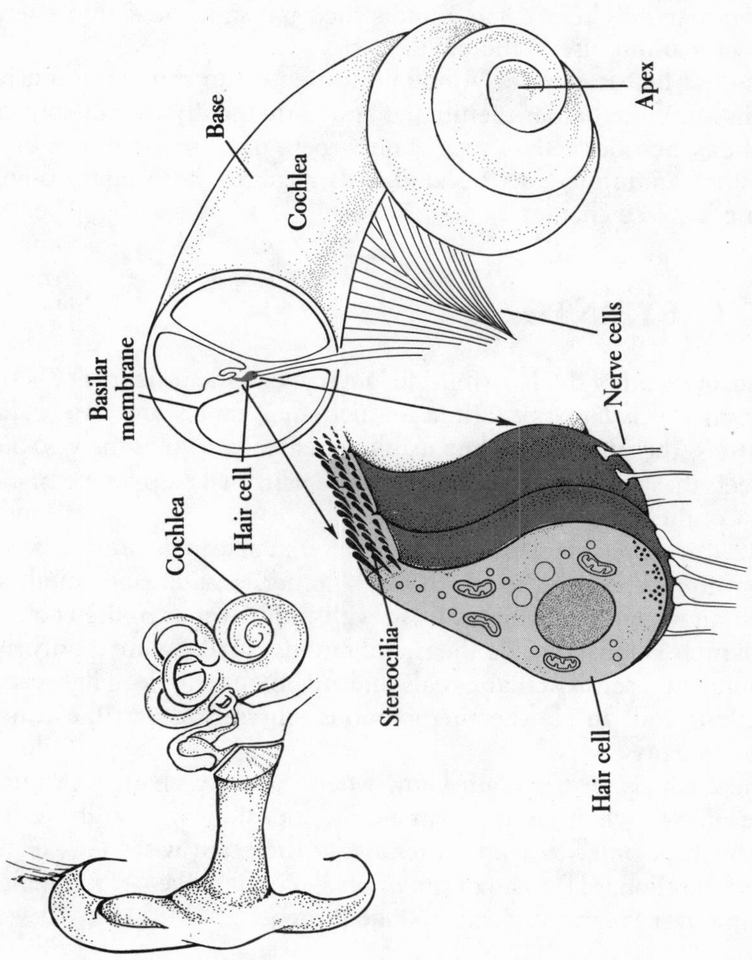

Hair cells (shown in gray) are suspended from a membrane in the spiral-shaped cochlea of the inner ear. Sound waves make the membrane vibrate. The hair cells can detect the motion because it causes the stereocilia to bend. These cells then stimulate the attached nerve cells. The membrane is most sensitive to high frequencies at the base of the spiral and to low frequencies at the apex of the spiral.

the membrane are sensitive to different sounds, however. The base, or closer end, is most sensitive to high-frequency sound. The top, which is the farthest end, has a greater sensitivity to sounds of low frequency.

The inner ear contains 10,000 to 15,000 hair cells that are arranged in rows. These rows of hair cells are in contact with a gelatinous membrane that sits on top. Sound waves lift the basilar membrane up and bend the hair cells against the jellylike tectorial membrane. That action triggers the release of a nerve transmitter substance at the base of the hair cells, which causes the auditory (or acoustic) nerve to fire. In a sense, the hair cells act much like circuits in a telephone system. When stimulated, they become electrically charged and in turn stimulate the auditory nerve. These nerve circuits then transmit the sound energy via electrical impulse to the brain.

A sound that is extremely loud and intense can throw the sensory cells right off the basilar membrane and permanently damage or rupture them. Sensory cells, a type of nerve cell, don't replace themselves when they are injured, so this kind of damage results in sensorineural hearing loss (see chapter 2).

THE LABYRINTH

The second part of the labyrinthine landscape of the inner ear contains the organs of balance: the three semicircular canals and two saclike structures, the utricle and the saccule. An area known as the vestibule connects these organs. Collectively, these parts make up the *vestibular system* of the ear.

The three pretzel-shaped, bony semicircular canals are tubes that are positioned at right angles to one another. Inside each canal is a membranous labyrinth that is filled with fluid. Just as in the cochlea, endolymph is found inside the membranous canals, while perilymph surrounds the semicircular canals and fills the vestibule. Highly sensitive hair cells inside the membranous labyrinth act as the canals' sensory organs.

These canals let the brain know when the body changes position. For example, when we turn our heads, the fluid shifts and the hair cells bend in order to send a message to the brain with news of this altered position. The canals themselves don't move—it's the fluid sloshing over the sensory cells that does the job.

Once changes in position occur, the fluid attempts to "catch up." More violent movement, such as spinning around in circles as part of a game or a dance, or riding on a carousel, may create a slight delay as the fluid tries to communicate the constant circular sensation to the brain. For example, imagine that you quickly carried a pan filled with water across a room and then, just as quickly, put it down. The liquid inside would continue to swirl around for a while. The same thing happens to the fluids in the inner ear.

This ability of the brain to constantly sense your position and maintain your balance depends on the smooth integration of your sense of vision, the reflex reactions of your muscles, and most important, the normal functioning of the labyrinth. Anyone who has ever suffered an inner-ear infection knows that such an ailment can produce the sensation of spinning, when in fact no motion is occurring. This false sense of motion is called *vertigo* (see chapter 8).

Another sensor inside the labyrinth is the utricle—one of two tiny sacs. It measures the body's response to the force of gravity and to linear acceleration. The hair cells inside the utricle respond to gravity when they are stimulated by thousands of tiny crystals, each one smaller than a grain of salt. These calcite crystals are called *otoconia*, the Greek word for "ear dust." These particles tumble onto the hair cells when you start to move, walk forward, slow your pace, speed up your step, or stop. The sensory hair cells in turn send the appropriate message to the brain. (Medical scientists still haven't determined the purpose of the other saclike sensor, the saccule.)

The human measuring device of gravity is the brain, which has its own set of standards for letting you know which end is up. If you are accustomed to standing on firm ground, for example, and then board a ship and encounter the rocking motion of a turbulent sea, you probably will become seasick. However, sailors and travelers who spend a great deal of time on the water usually develop "sea legs," or the ability to adjust to the constant motion of the sea without becoming sick (see chapter 8).

The sensory organs of the inner ear transmit their messages to the brain along two branches of nerve fibers—one from the cochlea and the other from the labyrinth—that together join to form the *auditory* (or *acoustic) nerve,* also called the eighth cranial nerve or cochleovestibular nerve.

Many nerves that provide sensation to the ear also serve other parts of the head and neck. When these nerves are stimulated, they can produce a sensation of pain coming from the ear when, in fact, that is not the case. This is known as *referred* pain.

Some typical sources of referred pain to the ear are temporomandibular joint (TMJ) pain, dental pain, sore throat, tonsillitis, inflamed sinuses, swollen glands in the throat, and even throat cancer.

Facial nerve. The facial nerve, which controls the movement of muscles that allow facial expressions, runs through the ear. Occasionally, an ailment that affects the ear may also interfere with the facial nerve, resulting in a facial paralysis such as Bell's palsy.

Bell's palsy affects an area of the facial nerve where the nerve canal is very narrow. If swelling from a minor viral infection, for example, occurs in this small area, the inflammation may pinch off the blood supply to the nerve. This may eventually result in the facial palsy.

2

Why Hearing Loss Occurs

About one in 10 Americans has some form of hearing impairment that affects the ability to understand speech and conduct a normal conversation, according to the National Institutes of Health (NIH). Of the estimated 28 million people in the United States with an actual hearing loss, it is thought that at least 10 million have diminished hearing as a result of exposure to excessive noise.

Since ancient times, certain occupations have been associated with work-related hearing loss—among them, metalworking and blacksmithing. And much of the hearing loss that did not arise from infection or disease was largely attributed to military or occupational exposure to noise. Now, hazardous noises and sounds that can cumulatively damage hearing are fast becoming ubiquitous, and affect everyone.

In 1990, amid growing concern over the increased incidence of hearing loss, a panel of experts convened by the National Institutes of Health reported that millions of Americans are exposed to excess noise at home, at work, and at play. As a result, irreversible damage to the hearing mechanism is occurring earlier and more frequently than in the past.

Hearing loss used to be a problem that most commonly affected older adults. This kind of age-related hearing loss, called *presbycusis*. is actually increasing as the elderly claim a larger share of the population. But researchers are now finding that many teenagers may be suffering some decline in hearing acuity as a result of the way they listen to popular music—especially through personal stereos and headphones.

A British researcher tested three groups of students who had been exposed to varying amounts of amplified music. Those who had logged an average of 2,000 hours were affected more than those who listened to the music for about 225 hours over the same period. The heavy listeners showed a 10 to 20 percent deterioration in their ability to hear certain sounds, especially when background noise was present.

Aging and excessive noise are among the more commonly recognized causes of hearing impairment, but there are others. Some hearing loss has a genetic basis and occurs in certain families. Infection, disease, and even the common cold can lead to complications that produce a temporary, and occasionally permanent, loss of hearing.

TYPES OF HEARING LOSS

There are two basic types of hearing loss: conductive and sensorineural. When the two types occur together, it is called a mixed hearing loss.

Conductive hearing loss disrupts the mechanical transmission of sound waves through the outer and middle ear. If sound energy cannot be conducted into the inner ear, it cannot be heard. Generally, most forms of conductive hearing loss can be treated or corrected.

Something as benign as earwax frequently produces temporary hearing loss. Foreign bodies in the ear, infection, and damage to the eardrum are among the other causes of conductive hearing loss. A fairly common condition called *otosclerosis* can stop the motion of one of the three tiny bones inside the middle ear, thus preventing the normal transmission of sound waves. Fortunately, this condition can be surgically corrected or alleviated by using a hearing aid.

A conductive hearing loss may be mild and clear up on its own, as in the case of aerotitis (barotrauma) resulting from a change of atmospheric pressure during an airplane trip. But when there is pain, a feeling of fullness in the ear, and some degree of hearing loss, medical attention is necessary.

Sensorineural hearing loss occurs when the sensory cells in the inner ear no longer can pick up incoming sound waves or transmit them to the brain. Damage to the cochlea, to the auditory nerve, or to the electrical pathways of the central nervous system can cause this kind

CAUSES OF CONDUCTIVE HEARING LOSS

1. Conditions that can block the outer ear canal:
   - Earwax
   - External otitis
   - Tumors
   - Foreign objects
   - Exostosis

2. Problems that can affect the eardrum:
   - Perforated eardrum
   - Infection

3. Common conditions affecting the middle ear:
   - Serous otitis media
   - Eustachian tube dysfunction
   - Chronic otitis media
   - Congenital abnormalities
   - Aerotitis (barotrauma)
   - Otosclerosis
   - Acute otitis media
   - Tumors

of impairment. Sensorineural hearing loss usually cannot be reversed, although treatment may be beneficial for certain conditions.

The death of sensory hair cells in the inner ear—the leading cause of sensorineural hearing loss—is usually associated with aging as a part of the condition called presbycusis. Long-term exposure to noise also has long been recognized as a cause of sensorineural hearing loss. A traumatic injury, such as a fractured skull or damage from a loud blast, can also destroy nerve cells in the cochlea. Certain drugs can be toxic to the inner ear. For example, aspirin, taken in large quantities—12

CAUSES OF SENSORINEURAL HEARING LOSS

- Aging (presbycusis)
- Infection
- Ménière's disease
- Drugs
- Noise
- Head trauma
- Tumors
- Genetic abnormality

CAUSES OF MIXED HEARING LOSS

- Chronic infections
- Surgery
- Congenital disorders
- Trauma to the head
- Tumors (rarely)

or more a day—can lead to tinnitus, or noise in the ear. Fluid balance problems in the inner ear (as in Ménière's disease) can also cause a sensorineural hearing loss.

Mixed hearing loss may arise from an infection that damages the eardrum and the trio of bones in the middle ear (the conductive portion of hearing). The infection then spreads into the inner ear, where it affects sensorineural hearing.

A tumor can also grow in the ear canal or in the middle ear, obstructing the flow of incoming sound by blocking the canal, interfering

Warning Signs of Hearing Loss

In our culture, hearing loss has been associated with aging, senility, loss of control, and even lack of intelligence. It's no wonder that many people have a tendency to deny any change in their hearing, unless the problem occurs suddenly. Unfortunately, it usually takes a while to become aware that your hearing may not be as good as it once was.

Some of the warning signs of adult hearing loss include:

- Asking people to repeat themselves
- Missing large parts of conversations held in noisy areas
- Difficulty hearing while talking on the telephone
- Finding it hard to understand dialogue at the movies or the theater
- Difficulty distinguishing other people's words when conversing in restaurants or while riding in a car
- Not understanding someone who is speaking loudly from another room. You can hear the person yelling, but you can't make out the words.

- An inability to understand conversation unless you're looking directly at the speaker's lips or face. Or, finding that every time you turn away, you miss what is being said.
- Having family members or friends often suggest that you should get your hearing checked
- Increasing isolation. Very often, a person who finds it difficult to hear stops socializing.

SIGNS IN CHILDREN

It may be very difficult to detect mild hearing loss in a child. Moreover, the warning signs of hearing impairment in children are often quite different from adult symptoms. Among the signs are:

- A high-risk pregnancy and delivery
- The child's poor response to sound as a newborn
- Delays in speech and language development
- Family history of hearing loss
- Behavior problems
- Frequent ear infections or persistent fluid in the middle ear
- Deteriorating grades in school

with eardrum motion, or damaging the three ossicles of the middle ear. A tumor that invades the inner ear can cause a sensorineural hearing loss, although this is a rare occurrence.

CONDUCTIVE HEARING LOSS IN THE OUTER EAR

Numerous conditions can affect the outer ear canal and eardrum. Some are caused by blockages, such as earwax or foreign bodies lodged in the ear, but others are the result of infections or hereditary conditions.

Earwax

Impacted earwax (cerumen) is a common cause of hearing loss. Wax that builds up in the ear canal or around the eardrum can prevent sound from reaching the middle ear.

Earwax is part of the outer ear's self-cleaning mechanism—it protects the ear from water, microorganisms, and dirt. Usually, if you maintain a hands-off policy in regard to earwax, you'll have no problems. However, there are some people who habitually "clean" their ears with cotton-tipped swabs or even with metal objects like bobby pins or safety pins. In trying to remove the earwax, they risk the very thing they are trying to correct—wax buildup. Although some of the wax is removed, most of it is actually pushed farther down the ear canal, where it accumulates and eventually blocks the ear. And if the cleaning object scrapes the delicate skin inside the ear canal, or scratches the eardrum, the small cut can lead to an infection.

Yet there are some people who refrain from these practices and still tend to produce excessive amounts of earwax. The wax accumulates and requires regular removal by a trained health-care provider. The buildup of wax may appear suddenly, producing a feeling of fullness or pressure, possibly pain, and causing some degree of hearing loss. At other times, a drop of water may lodge around the wax plug, causing it to swell and create a blockage.

Treatment. Once your health-care provider examines your ear and makes a diagnosis, the impacted earwax can be removed by means of irrigation, suction, or the use of a manual probe. As soon as the earwax is removed, your hearing should return to normal.

Ear-cleaning kits or drops to remove earwax safely at home are available over the counter. They can be effective if used properly. However, when accumulated wax produces an actual hearing loss, such self-treatment methods may provide little relief, and you should consult a physician.

People who wear hearing aids often require a yearly or twice-a-year removal of earwax by a health-care practitioner. The portion of the hearing aid that fits into the ear canal can block the natural migration of earwax out of this passageway and cause the cerumen to accumulate.

Foreign Bodies

Temporary hearing loss can occur when a foreign body lodges in the ear canal and obstructs it. Children who place small objects in their ears during play account for most of these cases, but adults occasionally require treatment for this problem as well. Small children often don't complain when they have a blockage in the ear canal. Sometimes the object isn't detected until the child receives a physical examination or develops an ear infection.

Treatment. Never attempt to remove a deeply lodged foreign object on your own, as you may tear the skin or push the object even deeper into the ear canal, possibly damaging the eardrum. A trained specialist with the appropriate instruments can remove it. In some cases, anesthesia may be necessary.

Swimmer's Ear (External Otitis)

An infection or fungus of the skin that lines the ear canal of the outer ear, swimmer's ear occurs more commonly in the summer months and in hot, humid climates. It can be a problem for swimmers and divers, but more often it affects people who use cotton-tipped swabs or other objects to remove wax or water from their ears. Occasionally, it can occur spontaneously, without any obvious cause.

The outer ear canal, which is open to the environment, is covered with microorganisms that normally reside on the skin. If the delicate skin lining the canal breaks, bacteria or fungi can enter the soft tissue below and cause an infection. The combination of a break in the normal skin barrier and the presence of moisture, microorganisms, and pollutants in water or swimming pools can lead to a case of swimmer's ear.

Mild itching and a feeling that the ear is plugged up are among the early symptoms. Scratching the itch with a swab or a fingernail further irritates the already sensitive skin and sets the stage for further infection. Severe pain and a discharge soon follow. Sometimes, hearing loss may accompany the infection as debris builds up in the ear canal, or the canal itself may swell shut and disrupt hearing.

Treatment. Your doctor will treat the infection by first gently cleaning debris from the ear canal. Ear drops that contain an antibiotic to combat infection, plus a steroid to reduce the swelling, are then applied. Drops that acidify the ear canal may be used, too. Among the drugs that may be prescribed are polymyxin B-neomycin-hydrocortisone (*Cortisporin Otic Suspension*). When swelling is excessive, the physician may place a piece of gauze or a compressed wick (*Merocel*) in the ear to allow the ear drops to come in contact with the entire length of the ear canal. Severe infections may be treated with oral antibiotics in addition to ear drops.

Usually, any severe pain disappears within two days of appropriate therapy. The infection normally clears up in seven to 10 days with regular use of the prescribed ear drops. (An alternate drug may be prescribed for those who are allergic to neomycin.)

During healing, care must be taken to keep the ear dry. Swimming must be avoided, and you must wear a shower cap or water-tight earplugs when taking a shower. Or you can coat a pair of cotton balls with petrolatum and insert them in your ears as an alternative to earplugs. Of course, these homemade earplugs should be discarded after each use.

To prevent swimmer's ear, you can buy over-the-counter ear drops that coat the inside of the ear canal. Apply them after swimming. A few drops of rubbing (isopropyl) alcohol can also be used after swimming or bathing to dry out the ear canal.

Malignant External Otitis

Diabetics or those whose immune systems have been weakened by an immunodeficiency disorder such as AIDS may develop an ear canal infection that is more serious than a simple case of swimmer's ear. This infection, usually caused by the pseudomonas bacterium, burrows deeper into the soft tissues of the ear canal. If left untreated, the infection can spread rapidly to the underlying tissues of the skull, eventually involving the brain itself.

Severe ear pain in a diabetic or someone with AIDS may be a primary early symptom of malignant external otitis. Treatment calls for emergency referral to a specialist who is an expert in the care of this disorder. Improper or delayed treatment can lead to a fatal outcome.

Surfer's Ear (Exostosis)

People who habitually swim in cold water—especially avid surfers—are at risk of developing *exostoses*, abnormal bony growths in the ear canal. This occurs when cool water repeatedly gets into the ear canal, and the canal responds to the cold temperature by setting down new layers of bone. Over time, little mounds of bone increase to the point where they may eventually block off the ear canal. These bony growths generally don't produce any symptoms unless water gets trapped behind them and causes a case of external otitis. Occasionally, these growths are seen in non-swimmers as well.

Rarely does surfer's ear progress far enough to block the ear canal and produce a conductive hearing loss. When there is such a blockage, a doctor can surgically remove the bony growths.

Underdeveloped Ears (Atresia)

When any part of the ear fails to develop fully during the normal nine-month growth period of a human fetus, the condition is known as *atresia*. In atresia, development of all or any of the tissues that make up the entire ear—the outer, middle, and inner ear—may not occur at all, or may be halted prematurely during fetal growth. Heredity, chromosomal abnormalities, and rubella are among the causes of atresia.

Hearing difficulties vary among people affected by atresia. In a sense, atresia can be compared to an unfinished house. The resulting structure works only as well as what already has been completed. An ear affected by atresia may be only mildly malformed and function normally, or it may be so severely malformed (with major portions of certain structures missing) that it doesn't function at all. Depending on the area that was most severely affected, this condition can produce a conductive, sensorineural, or mixed hearing loss.

Treatment. Atresia may involve one or both ears. When atresia affects the auricle, or shell-like portion of the outer ear, reconstructive surgery may be performed for cosmetic reasons. When the atresia affects *both* external ears and ear canals, it is usually recommended that surgery be performed on one ear canal during childhood to improve hearing. The other ear canal is usually reconstructed during the later teen years. However, cosmetic reconstruction of both auricles is carried out at about five or six years of age.

Ruptured Eardrum

A perforated eardrum may occur as a result of direct trauma, such as a puncture wound from a cotton-tipped swab or from pressure injuries caused by a nearby explosion or a blow over the ear. When the eardrum ruptures, the injury can interfere with the normal transmission of sound waves to the middle ear.

In addition to causing hearing loss, a ruptured eardrum can produce pain, bleeding, and a feeling of hollowness in the ear. (If dizziness accompanies these symptoms, see an otolaryngologist as soon as possible.)

Most simple perforations heal on their own as long as the injury is clean. Hearing also usually returns to normal. The size of the perforation influences the rate of healing; the smaller the hole, the quicker it is likely to heal. Large perforations may take weeks or even months to repair themselves.

Treatment. Some perforations, such as a rupture caused by poking a cotton-tipped applicator through the eardrum, may contaminate the area. Antibiotic drops are then prescribed to prevent infection. Sometimes the perforation can be covered with a paper "patch" to promote healing. (This can be done in the doctor's office.) Again, in most cases, the perforation heals naturally and full hearing capability returns. But if infection does set in, the chance of complete healing drops significantly.

If a perforated eardrum hasn't healed within a few months, an otolaryngologist can repair the hole. The doctor takes muscle-lining tissue, or fascia, from a nearby muscle to rebuild the eardrum. Immediate surgery also may be recommended when a person suffers a penetrating wound of the eardrum and debris and dirt have passed through the ear canal into the middle ear. (When there is suspected damage to the connections between the chain of ossicle bones in the middle ear, or in case of dizziness or severe sensorineural hearing loss, emergency surgery also may be necessary.)

Successful treatment of a perforated eardrum calls for keeping the affected ear dry and allowing no water to enter until the injury is completely healed. A piece of lambswool or cotton coated with petrolatum, or an earplug, can be placed in the ear to keep it dry during bathing.

CONDUCTIVE HEARING LOSS IN THE MIDDLE EAR

Middle ear problems range from infections to pressure changes, bone disorders, and cysts.

Middle-Ear Infection (Acute Otitis Media)

Otitis media—infection of the middle ear—is the most common cause of temporary and sometimes permanent hearing loss in young children. Otitis media usually affects children between the ages of five and eight; adults occasionally develop it as well. With prompt medical attention and the proper treatment, otitis media is not a serious problem. Delaying treatment, however, can cause the infection to spread to the inner ear.

When infectious bacterial or viral organisms enter the middle ear, they can produce an inflammation that results in *acute otitis media*. Very often, this infection occurs as a complication after a cold, influenza, or measles.

Pain, a feeling of pressure and blockage, and hearing loss in the affected ear are the typical symptoms of this disorder, which affects children more often than adults. Fever also may accompany the earache. Infants or toddlers who suddenly begin crying and tugging at one ear may be experiencing an earache associated with acute otitis media.

As the infection progresses, pus builds up in the middle-ear space, accompanied by severe pain. When a doctor examines the ear, the eardrum appears red and bulging from accumulated pus behind it. Sometimes, the pressure causes the eardrum to burst open and discharge the fluid into the ear canal. When this happens, the pressure is relieved and the pain almost immediately disappears.

Treatment. Oral antibiotics are prescribed to control the infection. Ear drops may be used as well if the ear is draining.

If the eardrum has ruptured, special care must be taken to avoid getting water into the child's affected ear. You may be advised to follow the time-tested practice of inserting a clean piece of cotton in the ear and then coating the outside with petrolatum before bathing the child.

In most cases, the rupture in the eardrum is small and usually heals on its own as the infection clears up. Occasionally, if the infection is especially virulent, it can cause a large perforation that may not heal, requiring further treatment. Also, severe or untreated infections can erode parts of the ossicles (the little bones of hearing), resulting in hearing loss.

Complications. Several complications may arise from a case of untreated acute otitis media. These include the possible spread of infection to the bony area behind the ear, into the inner ear, and directly to the facial nerve itself.

- *Mastoiditis*. This is an inflammation of the air-filled mastoid bone behind the ear. Only decades ago, thousands of children used to die annually from this infection. Mastoiditis is a rare condition today, thanks to antibiotics.

Pain, fever, malaise, hearing loss, and occasionally a discharge from the ear are symptoms of mastoiditis. The ear begins to protrude from the head, and the mastoid bone becomes very tender. Mastoiditis affects the whole body, much more than would a routine ear infection.

When a physician suspects mastoiditis, an otolaryngologist is usually consulted immediately. Treatment consists of a *myringotomy*, a small surgical incision in the eardrum to allow fluid to drain from the mastoid. Intravenous antibiotics are also used to control the infection. Surgery to remove infected areas of bone may be necessary if the response to antibiotic therapy is slow.

- *Labyrinthitis*. Sometimes the germ that causes acute otitis media may spread beyond the middle ear into the labyrinth of the inner ear and disrupt balance as well as hearing (see chapter 8).
- *Facial paralysis*. The facial nerve, which runs right through the ear, may become inflamed and swollen when acute otitis media is present. The result is an increasing loss of motion on one side of the face, such as an inability to close one eye or to smile. This loss of motion is usually resolved as the infection clears up.

Serous Otitis Media

Serous otitis media, or accumulated fluid in the middle ear, occurs when the eustachian tube (the tube running from the back to the middle of the nose to allow air into the middle ear) becomes swollen, inflamed, or doesn't work properly. Fluid then collects in the middle-ear space. It can remain there indefinitely, causing recurring ear infections, a conductive hearing loss, or both.

Children are most commonly affected by serous otitis media. Often there are no obvious symptoms, and routine hearing tests in school may reveal that a child has a hearing loss before parents are aware of it.

The eustachian tube may malfunction for any of several reasons: a cold, infected sinuses, throat infection, allergies, enlarged adenoids, and cholesteatomas (cysts). Cancer of the nasopharynx—the back of the nose—also may cause persistent middle-ear fluid in an adult. In adults over age 60, the soft tissue around the eustachian tube may become lax and tend to obstruct the tube, also resulting in the accumulation of fluid.

When the affected ear is examined, the eardrum lacks the motion it should normally have. Fluid also may be visible behind the eardrum. Depending on the thickness of the fluid in the middle ear, hearing loss may range from mild to severe, with a potential loss of as much as 40 decibels. This would make any normal conversation sound like a whisper. Fluid that is thicker, or more viscous, causes an even greater hearing loss.

Treatment. Initial treatment in children is with oral antibiotics. In the past, antihistamines and decongestants were given in the hope that these medications would help dry up the fluid. But several studies have shown that these drugs do not improve the condition. Steroids also have been used, but it's unclear whether they offer any benefit either.

When antibiotics alone are ineffective in clearing up the backed-up fluid, the physician may recommend the surgical insertion of tiny ventilation tubes through the eardrum into the middle ear. These tubes allow air to enter and exit the middle ear externally via the eardrum instead of through the back of the nose, thus bypassing the eustachian tube. Ventilation tubes can help prevent fluid from accumulating in the middle ear and restore hearing to its normal level. The tubes aren't visible unless someone peers down into the ear canal. Again, water must not get into the ear canal while the child is bathing.

Depending upon the type used, the tubes may drop out by themselves or, alternatively, need to be removed. It is not uncommon for fluid to recur after the tubes come out and the drum returns to normal. Occasionally, the eardrum doesn't heal on its own and further treatment is necessary.

Ventilation tubes are made from a variety of materials, including plastic and metal, and can safely remain in place for several months or even years. When the ventilation tube is finally removed, and if the eustachian tube is functioning adequately, fluid will not collect again and the middle ear will remain normally aerated.

Children who have had chronic infections of their adenoids and tonsils may have recurring serous otitis media. In that case, surgical removal of the adenoids may be recommended.

When an older adult has serous otitis media and there is no infection or tumor, the choice may be to live with the condition, especially if the hearing loss is mild. Otherwise, a ventilation tube can be placed

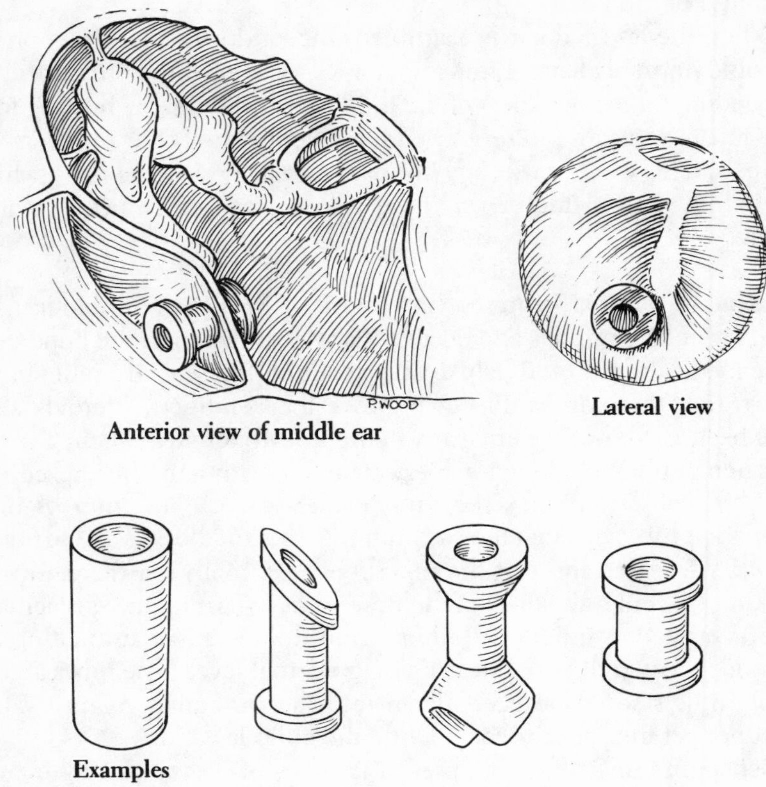

Ventilation tubes

in the adult's ear to aerate the middle ear and prevent the accumulation of fluid. A hearing aid may be recommended if the hearing loss is chronic and incapacitating.

Aerotitis (Barotrauma)

Sudden pressure changes in the atmosphere may occur while flying in an airplane or during a scuba dive. This condition is called *aerotitis*, also known as barotrauma. (There are several ways for airplane passengers and scuba divers to prevent aerotitis. These preventive measures are discussed in chapter 7.)

Under normal conditions of gravity, the pressure on the outside of the eardrum equals the pressure on the inside. Passengers in a descending airplane, however, have to increase pressure in the middle ear to equal the increase in outside pressure. This equilibration usually occurs when we yawn or swallow, causing the eustachian tube to open and allowing fresh air into the middle ear. But sometimes the eustachian tube does not function properly, and the pressure does not increase in the middle ear to equalize the outside pressure. Instead, the eardrum is pushed inward to compensate.

Pressure and pain result from this stretching of the eardrum. Occasionally, tiny blood vessels inside the eardrum may rupture, causing the eardrum to appear bruised. Sometimes, the eardrum itself may rupture, or fluid may collect in the middle ear.

Depending on the severity of the pressure injury, the problem may take hours or weeks to clear up on its own. Mild analgesics can help relieve the pain. Using a simple decongestant also may help decrease the sensation of pressure and help reopen the eustachian tube.

Most people who have an aerotitis injury don't suffer permanent hearing loss. However, a small group of people have a hearing system that cannot withstand the pressure change involved, and they risk more serious complications. Among these are bleeding from the ear or a leak of fluid from the inner ear that may cause dizziness or a sensorineural hearing loss.

When you suffer pain from a pressure change due to flying, it should not get any worse after you have landed. Seek medical attention if the condition progressively worsens or is accompanied by dizziness or hearing impairment.

Ear injury from pressure changes also can occur from scuba diving. Since the pressures involved with this activity are many times greater than with flying, the potential complications are much greater as well. Injury to the eardrum, disruption of the little bones of hearing (ossicles), and an inner-ear fluid leak all can result from scuba diving.

Otosclerosis

The most common cause of conductive hearing loss in young and middle-aged adults is otosclerosis, a bone disorder that affects the middle ear.

This condition causes an abnormal bony growth in the otic capsule, the extremely hard bone that houses the labyrinth of the inner ear. As the disease progresses, the compact bone is replaced with spongy bone and an increasing amount of bone deposits. This overgrowth of bone eventually extends to the edge of the oval window. Here, it can "lock" the stapes (the smallest of the ossicles) into place. When the stapes can no longer vibrate, sound waves cannot reach the inner ear and a loss of hearing results.

The cause of otosclerosis remains unknown, but the condition is probably genetic. The disorder affects women twice as often as men, and Caucasians have a tenfold greater likelihood of developing otosclerosis than do African-Americans. About one in 10 persons with this disorder develops hearing loss, and 30 to 40 percent of them will develop hearing loss in both ears. The hearing loss is gradual, progressing over periods of months to years.

Besides suffering a conductive hearing loss from fixation of the stapes, people with otosclerosis may develop a sensorineural hearing loss in the inner ear as well. It's not known why the inner ear undergoes this accelerated loss of hearing ability. One theory is that the growth of bone somehow releases harmful enzymes in the inner ear, eventually damaging the delicate hearing mechanism.

Treatment. Three choices are available to people with hearing loss due to otosclerosis: a period of observation, a hearing aid, or surgery.

In some cases, when the hearing loss is minimal, a specialist may recommend a course of observation. This usually involves an annual or biannual checkup to determine whether hearing has further declined. If there is a noticeable change in hearing in between checkups, it's important to alert the specialist.

A hearing aid may be prescribed for people who are having difficulty functioning with poorer hearing. Proper fitting for the aid should be carried out by an audiologist who has been specially trained to dispense hearing aids (see chapter 4).

The third treatment option is a surgical procedure called a stapedectomy. This procedure allows sound to enter the middle ear by bypassing the diseased bone. During this operation, part of the stapes bone is replaced with an artificial stapes. The otolaryngologist operates through the ear canal, going behind the eardrum to expose the middle-ear bones. One technique uses a laser or tiny drill to cut a hole in the foot plate of the stapes. The prosthesis is placed in the incision and hooked to the incus (the middle ossicle). In a second technique, the entire stapes is removed. A tissue graft (usually vein) is used to cover the inner ear and a prosthesis is placed between the incus and the graft. In both procedures, the eardrum is then put back into place.

When a skilled surgeon performs the stapedectomy, the success rate is 95 percent. The risk of damage to the inner ear—the sensorineural part of the hearing mechanism—is about 1 to 2 percent. Before deciding to undergo this surgery, discuss the benefits and risks of the procedure with your surgeon.

Cholesteatomas

A cholesteatoma is a cyst that develops from skin trapped in the middle ear. As all skin grows, the surface layers die. When this dead skin cannot be sloughed off, it builds up to form the cyst. As the dead skin accumulates, the size of the cyst increases, eventually damaging the surrounding middle-ear structures.

A cholesteatoma can even eat through the ossicles, thus causing a conductive hearing loss. If the expansion extends into the inner ear, it can produce dizziness and sensorineural hearing loss. In some severe cases, the cyst can press on the facial nerve and cause facial paralysis, affecting the ability to smile and to blink. And if the cyst becomes infected, persistent drainage from the ear may occur.

Some cholesteatomas are congenital, or present from birth, but most of these growths are acquired. The exact cause is not known, and this type of benign tumor can develop at any age.

Symptoms may include mild to severe hearing loss and the seepage of pus from the ear. When the inner ear is involved, dizziness may occur. Facial weakness or paralysis may be present if the facial nerve is affected.

Treatment. If infection is present, antibiotics are prescribed. Surgery to remove the cysts is recommended in almost all cases, unless the patient is in poor health.

SENSORINEURAL HEARING LOSS IN THE INNER EAR

The inner ear is the very core of the hearing apparatus. Any damage to this vital area can result in a hearing loss that may not be restorable. The outcome depends on the specific problem involved.

Presbycusis

Presbycusis, or age-related hearing loss, is the most common cause of hearing impairment in adults. Over the years, the sensory hair cells inside the cochlea of the inner ear die. The body does not replace these special cells. As the number of hair cells decreases, a point is eventually reached where hearing starts to decline. This gradual lessening of our ability to hear usually begins around age 60.

The hair cells that receive the higher-frequency tones, such as soprano pitches, are usually the first to deteriorate. Eventually, tones with a lower frequency, like those of everyday conversation, may be affected as well. Accompanying the loss of hearing is a declining ability to understand speech, especially when there is background noise. Early on, this may be the most troublesome complaint of people experiencing presbycusis.

Men tend to have a greater incidence of age-related hearing loss than do women. Studies have shown that beginning around age 10, females have consistently better hearing than their male counterparts, and that this difference continues well into old age. This gender difference is thought to be due to a man's increased exposure to occupational noise, such as working around heavy machinery and motors. As more women are exposed to noise at work, in the home, and in the overall environment, these numbers could change.

The term *presbycusis* refers to hearing as it is affected by the aging process alone. Another term often used—*sociocusis*—includes age-related hearing loss as well as exposure to potentially hazardous noise in the workplace and in everyday life. Indeed, it can be difficult for any specialist to say exactly how much of someone's hearing loss is due to physical aging or the auditory wear and tear of daily life.

Symptoms. An early symptom of age-related hearing loss is difficulty in understanding (rather than not hearing) speech when people talk. This is especially true when an older person misses words in a conversation taking place in a noisy restaurant, for example, or in a crowded room. The voices of women and children may also be harder to hear than the deeper tones of men. High-pitched sounds, like the chirping of birds, may not be audible at all.

Older adults with presbycusis often experience a phenomenon called *recruitment,* in which they perceive louder incoming sounds as *too* loud. For instance, raising your voice to speak to someone with presbycusis may prompt the common response "Don't shout, I'm not deaf."

As a result, people with recruitment may have trouble with hearing aids, especially if their units aren't properly fitted and adjusted.

Treatment. There's no easy way to relieve age-related hearing loss. In the early stages, it's possible to supplement a good amount of hearing with visual cues and lipreading (see chapter 9).

Eventually, as frustration builds, a person with age-related hearing loss may decide to wear a hearing aid or look into other assistive listening devices that may be helpful. It has been estimated that up to 40 percent of people over age 60 could benefit from some device to improve their hearing. But according to the results of a National Health interview survey, up to 58 percent of people over age 65 reported some hearing impairment, yet only 8 percent used a hearing aid. Even today, with the technological advances in hearing aids, too many older adults consider hearing loss to be an uncorrectable condition that comes with aging. Although people rarely go completely deaf from presbycusis, it can be a major impediment in personal communication.

Noise-Induced Hearing Loss

Because noise isn't an obvious pollutant, its harmful effects on hearing—and health—are rarely appreciated until it's too late. With enough exposure to potentially hazardous sounds, the auditory structures of the inner ear eventually suffer permanent damage.

Noise appears to cause chemical changes and physical damage to the delicate hair cells of the inner ear as well as swelling of nerve fiber endings inside the cochlea. Early on, the noise damages the closer end, or the base, of the cochlea—the area that is most sensitive to high-frequency sound. The amount of damage to your ears depends on the loudness of the noise, how long it lasts, and your individual sensitivity.

Overexposure to excessive noise produces a *temporary threshold shift (TTS)*, a brief change in hearing that may last for hours or days. When TTS occurs, sounds appear to be muffled. There may be a sensation of fullness in the ear and some ringing or buzzing.

An example of temporary threshold shift: People who work in a noisy environment often turn up the volume on their car radios while driving home at the end of the workday. When they turn on the radio the next morning, the higher volume is irritatingly loud and they immediately turn it down. The need to listen at a lower volume indicates that the hair cells in the inner ear had sustained damage and then underwent some repair overnight.

Rock concertgoers are at special risk of developing TTS. It's not unusual to find members of the audience shouting at one another outside the concert hall afterward—not out of anger, but because they can't hear very well. Some people may become very sensitive to noise after an especially loud concert and avoid listening to any music until their hearing undergoes the early phase of repair.

Recovery and prevention. There are two phases of recovery from exposure to loud noise. First, a rapid phase of repair takes place within the first day of noise injury. At this time, the broken and twisted hair cells actually repair themselves and will appear normal under a microscope. A slow repair process then takes place, which may take as long as a month.

With repeated exposure, or one severe exposure, the inner ear loses its ability to recover and undergoes a *permanent threshold shift* (PTS). In this irreversible condition, the hair cells rupture or die and permanent hearing loss follows. Determining the point at which damage from noise exposure will occur is difficult because some people are much more sensitive to noise than others.

The only way to avoid noise-induced hearing loss is by preventing it in the first place. Prevention hinges on two basic elements: (1) taking measures to control noise in your immediate environment, and (2) using personal hearing protection devices when you must be around noise. If you suspect that you have already developed noise-induced hearing loss, consult a hearing specialist as soon as possible.

For more information on preventing noise-induced hearing loss, see chapter 7.

Acoustic Trauma

Exposure to an explosion, or to any extremely loud noise, may damage the ear and result in a sensorineural hearing loss. This type of sound may be brief but of such intensity that it can virtually tear apart the sensory structures of the auditory portion of the inner ear.

This type of acute acoustic trauma usually produces a sudden change in hearing ability immediately after the exposure. Dizziness may occur, and the eardrum may rupture from the trauma. The ear that is closest to the source of the noise may be more damaged than the other ear. But if both ears are exposed equally, then both are likely to suffer a similar hearing loss.

Beyond the Ear: The Effects of Noise on Health

The effect of noise on our general health remains unknown, but preliminary research into this area has made one thing apparent: Noise can make you sick.

Studies have shown that noise can quicken the heart rate, increase blood pressure, and elevate blood cholesterol levels. Although there are no conclusive findings in terms of how noise affects the heart and blood vessels, its major effect on the cardiovascular system appears to be an elevation of blood pressure.

Scientists at Johns Hopkins University found that noise and carbon monoxide together may worsen the effects of noise exposure. In one study, laboratory animals were given the equivalent amount of carbon monoxide that is inhaled when a person smokes a cigarette. The animals then were exposed to noise levels that corresponded to those experienced by first-row spectators at an indoor rock concert. After just one exposure to this noise, the animals suffered a permanent hearing loss of 20 decibels. Researchers surmise that carbon monoxide may impede the flow of oxygen to the inner ear, which may require an increased supply of oxygen in response to higher noise levels. This is not yet proven, however.

Noise also may be damaging to the auditory system of the developing fetus. For this reason, pregnant women should avoid any exposure to excessive noise. (There is no evidence, however, that ultrasound causes any damage to the developing fetus.)

In children, noise may have a negative effect on reading ability. Elementary students who lived on the lower floors of a building close to a noisy expressway were found to have greater impairment in reading levels than children living on the higher floors.

The skills of children whose schools were located near a major airport were compared with students from schools in quieter areas. The children in the noisier environment had more difficulty in performing cognitive tasks.

Depending on the loudness of the noise, there may be partial or total recovery after several hours or days. If dizziness occurs, hearing does not return to normal, or the characteristic ringing of tinnitus persists, consult a hearing specialist as soon as possible.

Ménière's Disease

Ménière's disease, a condition in which fluid in the inner ear puts increased pressure on the walls of the labyrinth, can produce a fluctuating sensorineural hearing loss. Episodes of vertigo, or loss of balance, and tinnitus also accompany Ménière's disease (see chapter 8).

Ototoxic Drugs

Several commonly used medications can produce adverse effects on the inner ear and cause a temporary or permanent hearing loss. Among these are some analgesics, antibiotics, diuretics, and some chemotherapy drugs.

- *Aspirin*. The salicylate family of medications—which includes aspirin (acetylsalicylic acid)—is the most widely used group of medications in the United States. Taking excessive quantities of this analgesic (more than 12 aspirin tablets daily for longer than a few days; some people are more sensitive) can cause tinnitus, or a constant ringing in the ears, and hearing loss. Fortunately, the tinnitus and hearing loss usually clear up when aspirin use is decreased or stopped.
- *Aminoglycoside antibiotics*. The aminoglycoside antibiotics—including amikacin, gentamicin, kanamycin, neomycin, streptomycin, and tobramycin—are used to fight serious infections. In certain dosages, however, these drugs may have harmful side effects on the inner ear and kidneys.

  Some of the aminoglycosides are more toxic to the auditory (hearing) portion of the inner ear and actually damage the hair cells, causing a sensorineural hearing loss. Other aminoglycosides inflict their damage mostly on the vestibular (balance) system and can cause a permanent feeling of imbalance.

  Studies of laboratory animals have shown that overuse of aminoglycoside antibiotics may also increase the likelihood that the patient's hearing may be permanently injured by loud noises.

  When a physician carefully monitors the dose of aminoglycosides, sensorineural hearing loss usually can be prevented. Occasional cases of hearing loss can occur despite proper monitoring, however, for reasons that are not well understood.

- *Diuretics.* High doses of diuretics such as ethacrynic acid (*Edecrin*) and furosemide (*Lasix, Myrosemide*), used in the treatment of hypertension, can produce temporary hearing loss.
- *Quinine.* Quinine and quinine-like quinidine have been associated with sensorineural hearing loss after long-term use, or with ingestion during pregnancy. Quinine is used to treat malaria; quinidine is used to treat irregular heartbeat.
- *Beta-blockers.* Beta-blockers such as metoprolol and propanolol can cause tinnitus and a mild hearing loss.
- *Chemotherapy drugs.* Chemotherapeutic drugs used in the treatment of cancer—particularly cisplatin (Platinol)—can be highly toxic to the inner ear. For this reason, people who receive cisplatin need to be checked for hearing loss before and after completing their chemotherapy. Researchers have discovered that a drug called phosphomycin has alleviated the ototoxicity of cisplatin, at least in some small clinical trials. However, large clinical studies of phosphomycin's effectiveness in this regard have not yet been conducted.

In cases when two different drugs are administered together, the toxic effect may sometimes be more severe than if either were used alone. For instance, an aminoglycoside antibiotic in combination with a furosemide diuretic has greater potential to cause damage to hearing.

Treatment. When medication is toxic to the ear, it produces such signs and symptoms as tinnitus (ringing), vertigo (imbalance), and hearing loss. The only way to avoid hearing loss from these drugs is through prevention.

Many of these drugs are given to very sick people, and the doctors who prescribe them will carefully monitor the level of medication in the blood. It is also important that doctors frequently ask patients who are on these drugs if they are experiencing any symptoms that would point to the early signs of hearing loss.

Autoimmune Hearing Loss

People with autoimmune diseases such as lupus erythematosus or rheumatoid arthritis may develop a sensorineural hearing loss that rapidly progresses over a period of weeks or months. (This same pattern

Sudden Hearing Loss

Although hearing loss usually tends to develop gradually, there are instances in which it can occur abruptly: Within seconds or over a few hours, one loses the ability to hear.

Sudden hearing loss may be the result of earwax that has accumulated around the eardrum, for example. Middle-ear fluid or infection can also cause a sudden change in hearing. A viral infection and an alteration in blood flow to the inner ear (such as occurs with a small stroke) may be other causes of sudden hearing loss.

Typically, sudden hearing loss occurs in one ear, although in rare cases it can affect hearing on both sides. Vague symptoms may accompany the loss, including a ringing in the ears and a brief episode of vertigo. Diagnostic testing will help determine whether this sudden impairment of hearing is mild, moderate, or severe, and will aid the specialist in choosing treatment.

A person with sudden mild hearing loss usually experiences a spontaneous recovery within three to six weeks, whether or not treatment is sought or the problem is allowed to heal on its own. Moderate hearing loss, in which a person may lose 20 to 60 decibels of hearing ability, has a spontaneous recovery rate of about 30 percent. When sudden hearing loss is severe—greater than 60 decibels—some people may fully recover, but most must live with impaired hearing even after treatment.

Some studies have shown that the chance of recovery improves if the affected person is seen by a doctor within seven days of the onset of the problem. Treatment hinges on the administration of high doses of steroids—60 milligrams of prednisone a day—tapered over a two-week period. Other treatments have been used for sudden hearing loss, but only steroids have shown success, at least in some studies.

of hearing loss may also occur in people who have no other evidence of autoimmune disease.)

The hearing loss seems to be the direct result of the autoimmune disease, in which the body attacks its own tissues. The immune system manufactures antibodies to defend itself against antigens, or foreign invaders. But instead of attacking foreign antigens, some of the antibodies attack the tissues of the inner ear.

Women are more likely to develop autoimmune hearing loss—usually between the ages of 20 and 50. Special blood tests may be used to diagnose this disorder, but these difficult tests are still under investigation.

Treatment consists of high doses of steroids for a long period of time, or the use of chemotherapy drugs. Because these medications can cause serious side effects, the patient must be under the close supervision of a physician.

Perilymph Fistulas

Trauma is usually responsible for causing a fistula, which allows leakage of perilymphatic fluid into the area surrounding the round or oval windows of the inner ear. When fluid leaks from the inner ear to the middle ear, hearing loss or imbalance can occur.

Sneezing, coughing, and vigorous nose-blowing have been known to produce a perilymphatic fistula. However, the more common causes are head injuries, pressure changes from flying or scuba diving, and excessive straining when lifting weights.

Among the symptoms of a fistula are sudden or fluctuating hearing loss, a feeling of fullness in the ear, episodes of imbalance, and tinnitus.

Because the fistula cannot be seen, diagnosis is made partially on the basis of the patient's medical history or on the events that preceded the symptoms. A simple pressure and balance test also may be used to help confirm the presence of a fistula. Unfortunately, there are at present no clinically proven tests that can absolutely diagnose this condition in a high percentage of cases.

Treatment. Bed rest is the first line of treatment. In most cases, a fistula heals spontaneously. But if the hearing loss progresses or the dizziness persists, surgery to close the leaking area may be recommended. Surgery helps keep the hearing loss from progressing any further and usually arrests the dizziness.

Genetic and Congenital Hearing Loss in Children

Children may suffer sensorineural hearing loss in the womb, at birth, or during their growing years, from both genetic or acquired causes.

Genetic (hereditary) hearing loss. Children who are born to parents with a family history of deafness may be at high risk of having a hearing impairment. Hereditary conditions arise from defects in genes that may influence the developing hearing mechanism in the fetus.

These disorders, or *syndromes*, can cause abnormalities in the outer, middle, or inner ear. One such disorder, Waardenburg's syndrome, accounts for an estimated 2 to 3 percent of the 1 million cases of congenital deafness in the United States. In addition to hearing loss, Waardenburg's syndrome is often characterized by widely spaced eyes, a different color in each eye, and a white forelock of hair.

Children born with another disorder, Usher's syndrome, often develop vestibular (balance) problems along with hearing loss. In later childhood, they may suffer from a visual disturbance called retinitis pigmentosa, in which the retina of the eye disintegrates, leading to blindness.

Chromosomal errors also may occur. Instead of having the normal 23 pairs of chromosomes, the embryo has one extra or missing chromosome. The most common chromosomal abnormality is Down's syndrome, or Trisomy 21, which causes mental retardation and other symptoms in newborns. The abnormalities that can affect fetal hearing as well as other major organs are Trisomy 13 (Patau syndrome) and Trisomy 18 (Edwards's syndrome). Fortunately, both of these conditions are rare.

Congenital hearing loss. In many cases, congenital hearing loss isn't due to genetic causes but rather occurs as a result of infection, drugs taken during pregnancy, or injury to the fetus at birth.

One example is when a woman becomes infected with rubella (German measles) during the first three months of pregnancy. The infection can cause an irreversible hearing loss in the fetus. Although rubella is generally a mild illness in adults, it can produce other serious fetal complications, including mental retardation, cardiac defects, and cataracts. However, hearing loss is the most common result of congenital rubella.

Infection with such viruses as cytomegalovirus, herpes, or syphilis during pregnancy also increases the risk of acquired hearing loss in a newborn.

Some drugs ingested during pregnancy may be toxic to the developing hearing mechanism. Although scientists don't yet know the effects of most drugs on the developing ear of the fetus, thalidomide and quinine have been documented to have unfortunate results. When many pregnant women (mostly in Europe) took thalidomide back in the late 1950s, they bore infants with severe defects of the ear as well as deformed arms and legs. Quinine also carries a risk of producing deafness in both ears of an infant.

Infants who are born prematurely, have low birth weights, or suffer a lack of oxygen from prolonged childbirth or from interference with the blood supply during delivery are also at a higher risk of hearing impairment.

MIXED HEARING LOSS: THE MIDDLE AND INNER EAR

Infections that begin in the middle ear can spread and extend into the inner ear, causing hearing problems.

Chronic Otitis Media

When a middle-ear infection persists over a long period of time, or keeps recurring, the condition is often called *chronic otitis media*. If left untreated, it can damage the eardrum and the ossicles and cause a conductive hearing loss. The infection also can damage the inner ear and produce a sensorineural hearing loss.

Chronic otitis media may have such symptoms as drainage from the ear, pain, and hearing loss.

Treatment. If you have chronic otitis media, your doctor will prescribe antibiotics for the infection. If the medication doesn't resolve the problem, surgery is usually recommended. Any perforations in the eardrum can be surgically repaired, and damaged hearing bones can be reconstructed. Although the conductive part of the hearing loss can often be corrected, any sensorineural hearing loss cannot be reversed.

Trauma

Injury or trauma to the ear or to the head can cause hearing loss. Depending on which part of the hearing mechanism is affected, the hearing loss may be conductive or sensorineural.

A fall, a blow to the head, even scraping the ear canal or eardrum with a cotton-tipped applicator are among the various causes of trauma to the ear that may produce a conductive hearing loss. Acoustic trauma is a type of sensorineural hearing loss that can follow a serious blow to the ear or a skull fracture. It can also occur in response to an explosive noise or blast.

Physical trauma to the outer ear, such as a cut or scrape, may cause an infection as well. Dirt may enter the wound, or bacteria on the skin may invade the wound to cause an infection. If a cut of the outer ear is severe or appears swollen, red, or is painful, seek medical care. Antibiotic drops and/or oral antibiotics may be prescribed. Usually, contact with water must be avoided until the injury is fully healed.

When there is conductive hearing loss following physical trauma, hearing usually returns on its own. If there has been a tear in the eardrum, for example, the tissue usually repairs itself. When the ossicles have been disrupted by trauma, they may heal and scar in such a way that this conductive sound mechanism is restored to near-normal. If damage to the eardrum or ossicles causes a permanent problem, surgery can usually correct it.

Damage to the inner ear from trauma sometimes can partially heal on its own. If the hearing loss is severe, however, a hearing aid may be necessary.

Tumors

A variety of tumors can grow in the ear and cause hearing loss, pain, or fluid drainage. A benign tumor called an acoustic neuroma is the most common tumor affecting the ear. Other benign tumors are the glomus tympanicum (chemodectoma), the glomus jugulare, and the cholesteatoma, a skin cyst that was discussed previously in this chapter.

Acoustic neuroma. This small tumor grows slowly in the inner ear canal on the balance (vestibular) branch of the eighth cranial nerve. The fibers of this nerve carry information about hearing and balance from the inner ear to the brain. Because an acoustic neuroma presses against the hearing (auditory) branch of the nerve, it produces hearing loss as an early symptom. Typically, a person will begin to have difficulty in discrimination, or understanding what other people are saying.

An acoustic neuroma is not malignant and won't spread to other parts of the body, but it can enlarge and eventually cause damage by placing pressure on neighboring structures. If neglected, an acoustic neuroma can push into the brain cavity and cause severe, life-threatening problems.

Some hearing loss (occasionally sudden) and tinnitus, or ringing in the ears, may be the only early symptoms. Eventually the tumor may cause some imbalance problems, but its slow growth may make them hardly noticeable. When an acoustic neuroma gets larger, it may produce such symptoms as numbness in the face and difficulty in swallowing.

Treatment. If your doctor suspects an acoustic neuroma, the first step is a physical examination of the ear and a hearing test. An evoked response audiogram (see chapter 3) or a magnetic resonance imaging (MRI) scan with contrast media may be ordered to confirm the diagnosis.

Treatment of the neuroma will depend on your age. If the tumor is small and you are over 65 or seriously ill, your doctor may recommend observation and follow-up with a series of MRI scans to determine whether the tumor is still growing or has remained stable in size.

If you are under 65, if you are trying to preserve your remaining hearing, or if you have a large growing tumor, surgery may be recommended. An otolaryngologist usually teams up with a neurosurgeon to remove the neuroma.

The most common complication of surgery is injury to the facial nerve. To reduce this risk, your surgeons will use special equipment to monitor the electrical activity of your hearing and your facial nerve during the procedure.

Some medical centers offer radiation therapy for acoustic neuromas, but this type of treatment remains experimental and unproven. It is also possible that the radiation may carry more complications than surgical treatment.

Glomus tympanicum and glomus jugulare. These vascular tumors usually produce a conductive hearing loss, although they can also affect sensorineural hearing.

Because both tumors have a very rich blood supply, they are often accompanied by a pulsating form of tinnitus that matches the rhythmic beating of the heart. A doctor who examines the ear can sometimes see a pulsating reddish mass behind the eardrum.

Depending on the size of the glomus tumor, and your age and

general health, your doctor may recommend observation, radiation therapy, or surgical removal.

Malignant tumors. Squamous cell carcinoma, adenocarcinoma, and metastatic cancers of the breast, lung, and kidney can invade the temporal bone, which houses the ear structure. These tumors are rare, however. When they do occur, the growths can produce hearing loss, dizziness, or pain in the ear. Treatment is with radiation or surgery, or both.

CENTRAL HEARING LOSS

Central hearing loss is quite different from conductive and sensorineural impairment. In this condition, the hearing mechanism is normal, but an injury to the brain or to the pathways of the central nervous system keeps the message from getting through.

PSYCHOGENIC HEARING LOSS

Psychogenic hearing loss affects the mind, not the hearing mechanism. The physical apparatus of the ear functions normally, but for unknown reasons—physical or psychological—the affected person doesn't process the information so that it can be heard and understood.

People with a psychogenic hearing loss seem unaware of sounds or words in their immediate environment. However, a hearing specialist can conduct tests (called evoked response audiometry) to confirm that the appropriate nerve signals are being conducted through the auditory (acoustic) nerve. When the diagnosis indicates a psychogenic disorder, a hearing specialist usually will recommend consultation with a psychiatrist.

While those individuals with a psychogenic hearing loss may have psychological blocks to hearing, others actually may pretend to be deaf but have perfectly normal hearing. An audiologist can detect this fact by using certain tests that make it difficult for anyone to pretend otherwise.

3

Testing and Diagnosis of Hearing Problems

Discovery of a hearing loss usually occurs when the problem begins to interfere with normal communication. It can happen at any age:

- A five-month-old infant fails to respond to sounds the way his older brothers did at the same age. His parents take him to their pediatrician, who recommends a medical examination by a pediatric hearing specialist. A hearing evaluation is ordered, and it reveals a moderate sensorineural hearing impairment.

  The parents learn that their child can be expected to keep up with children of the same age in school, but his speech and language development may take longer. Through an audiologist, they make arrangments to fit the child with a hearing aid and schedule classes in special speech-language therapy.
- A 59-year-old taxi dispatcher is accustomed to hearing family members tell him that he turns up the volume on the television so loud that it annoys others in the room. At work, surrounded by a bank of loudly ringing telephones and squawking receivers, he quickly responds to calls from the fleet of cabs he has dispatched for years.

  He is disturbed to discover that lately he has been missing some incoming information and occasionally has sent a driver to the wrong address. Fearful of losing his job, he visits his doctor, who

FIVE-MINUTE HEARING TEST

Simply mark the column that best describes how often you experience each situation or feeling.

	Almost always	Half the time	Occasionally	Never
1. I have a problem hearing over the telephone.				
2. I have trouble following the conversation when two or more people are talking at the same time.				
3. People complain that I turn the TV volume too high.				
4. I have to strain to understand conversations.				
5. I miss hearing some common sounds like the phone or doorbell ringing.				
6. I have trouble hearing conversations in a noisy background such as a party.				
7. I get confused about where sounds come from.				
8. I misunderstand some words in a sentence and need to ask people to repeat themselves.				
9. I especially have trouble understanding the speech of women and children.				
10. I have worked in noisy environments (assembly lines, jackhammers, jet engines, etc.).				
11. Many people I talk to seem to mumble (or don't speak clearly).				
12. People get annoyed because I misunderstand what they say.				

13. I misunderstand what others are saying and make inappropriate responses.				
14. I avoid social activities because I cannot hear well and fear I'll reply improperly.				
To be answered by a family member or friend: **15.** Do you think this person has a hearing loss?				

Scoring

To calculate your score, give yourself three points for every time you checked the "Almost always" column, two for every "Half the time," one for every "Occasionally," and zero for every "Never." If you have a blood relative who has a hearing loss, add another three points. Then total your points.

The American Academy of Otolaryngology—Head and Neck Surgery recommends the following:

- 0 to 5—Your hearing is fine. No action is required.
- 6 to 9—Suggest you see an ear, nose, and throat (ENT) specialist.
- 10 and above—Strongly recommend you see an ear physician.

Source: Reprinted by permission of the American Academy of Otolaryngology—Head and Neck Surgery, Inc., Washington, DC.

---

in turn refers him to a hearing specialist. Following testing and diagnosis, the dispatcher is found to have a moderate hearing loss that can be easily corrected by using a hearing aid.

- A 76-year-old retired teacher who enjoys attending bridge parties at the homes of her friends and having guests in for tea has been noticing that she has difficulty hearing telephone conversations. After seeing an ear specialist, she now has an amplifying device on her telephone. The physician sees no need to prescribe a hearing aid for her mild age-related hearing loss, although it may be necessary in the future.

In these three cases, the observant parents gave their baby a good start on getting the help he needed, and the dispatcher and the retiree were willing to admit there was a problem and to seek help. By getting treatment for these different types of hearing loss, they have improved their quality of life and retained their connection with the world around them.

When there is any question that your ability to hear is not normal, or you suspect that your child's hearing is impaired, it's important to get an evaluation by a physician who specializes in disorders of the ear.

Time lost in seeking a diagnosis is crucial, especially for infants unable to hear, for they are losing the opportunity to repeat and imitate words. The sooner such children receive a hearing aid or instruction in speech, the greater the chance they can overcome a speech or language deficit. Children who are found to be deaf present special problems (see chapter 9).

A HEARING SELF-TEST

Most of us can't help but notice a sudden change in our hearing, but a gradual change may occur so subtly that it's hardly apparent.

The American Academy of Otolaryngology has put together a brief self-examination quiz that was field-tested on 71 older adults in five U.S. cities. Those whose scores pointed to hearing problems were confirmed on an audiogram test as having a hearing impairment.

The self-test is found on pages 52–53.

SEEING A SPECIALIST: WHAT TO EXPECT

Some physicians specialize in hearing disorders: the otolaryngologist, or ear, nose, and throat specialist, and the otologist, who is a subspecialist with intense training in ear problems.

There is a widely held but erroneous belief that everyone who goes for a hearing evaluation receives the same prescription: a hearing aid. But it's impossible for a doctor to simply prescribe the same solution for all patients: The type and degree of hearing loss varies with each individual, and so does the treatment.

When you visit a hearing specialist for the first time, he or she will ask you a series of questions. Your answers are important for the diagnosis of your problem. You will be asked:

- How would you describe your complaint?
- Do you have problems hearing from one ear in particular?
- Do you think the hearing in both of your ears is about the same?
- How long have you had the problem?

- Did it occur suddenly or gradually, so that you hardly recognized it?
- When do you have trouble hearing—on the phone, when there's background noise, or in all conversations, wherever they take place?
- How is this problem with hearing affecting you—professionally, personally, socially?
- Do you have tinnitus, pain, or vertigo?

These questions, along with others about your age, occupation, medical history, family history of illness, and other pertinent information, including any medications you use, are a key part of the office visit. Taken together, they make up your total medical history, which allows the doctor to review the possible causes of your disorder and determine how any hearing loss is affecting the quality of your life.

A physical examination—which includes a careful inspection of your nose, mouth, and throat structures as well as your ears—follows. The doctor peers into the external portion of the ear and into the ear canal with an instrument called an otoscope. Using a bright light to illuminate the ear canal, the doctor inspects this narrow passage, taking care to note whether there are any obstructions of the ear canal, congenital malformations, or growths that may be due to a tumor.

Looking farther down the canal, the specialist observes the condition of the tympanic membrane (eardrum) for signs of inflammation, perforation, bulging retraction, or the presence of fluid behind it.

The otolaryngologist also examines the nose and the nasopharynx (the back of the nose where the eustachian tube drains). If allergies or congestion are present, the inflammation could affect the functioning of this tube. While inspecting the nasopharynx, the doctor also checks the area for any signs of tumor growth.

The final step is to test your hearing. An ear specialist usually performs a few basic tests in the office. Some doctors may use otoscopes designed to emit tones in the ear, but tuning forks are usually the instruments used to roughly determine whether you have a conductive or a sensorineural hearing loss. Later, additional hearing tests administered by a trained audiologist will define and quantify the actual degree of your hearing loss.

After the physical examination, the office tests, and an audiological evaluation, the physician usually has enough information to make a final diagnosis and design the best treatment for your particular needs.

Tuning Fork Tests

Tuning forks are simple but important basic testing devices that enable the ear specialist to distinguish one type of hearing loss from another.

Although there are tuning forks of various frequencies, the one that is most commonly used by a hearing specialist has a frequency of 512 hertz—the equivalent of the middle C tone on the piano. (When you strike this key, the piano wires vibrate about 512 times per second.) This frequency is at the lower end of the human speech range, which runs from 500 to 2,000 hertz. Tuning forks of other frequencies correspond to octaves of C that are higher or lower on the scale.

The two basic tuning fork tests are the Weber test and the Rinne test.

Weber test. The Weber test helps the doctor to find out whether your hearing is more sensitive in one ear than in the other. In this test, the vibrations from the tuning fork travel through the bone of the skull and stimulate the auditory nerve.

After striking the tuning fork against a surface to set it vibrating, the physician first places the stem of this device in the center of your forehead. As the vibrating fork is pressed against the bone, you will be asked which ear can hear the sound the loudest.

If the tone remains in the middle, it means that both ears are hearing equally as well. But if the sound goes only to the left or the right ear, it can indicate either a conductive hearing loss in the ear it travels to or a sensorineural hearing loss in the other ear. To tell which one it is, the Rinne test is performed.

Rinne test. This test is used to compare air conduction with bone conduction in the ear. (Sound waves enter the ear as vibrations of air. Then, as they travel from the outer ear to the middle ear, they change into vibrations in the bone.)

In the bone conduction part of the test, the base of the vibrating tuning fork is held against the mastoid bone behind one ear while a distracting sound is introduced into the other ear. Next, the vibrating tines of the fork are held a few inches away from the ear to determine the ear's air-conduction ability. These actions may be repeated until you are certain whether you are hearing the sound louder by means of air or behind your ear, through the bone.

If you are better able to hear the tone behind the ear, you may have

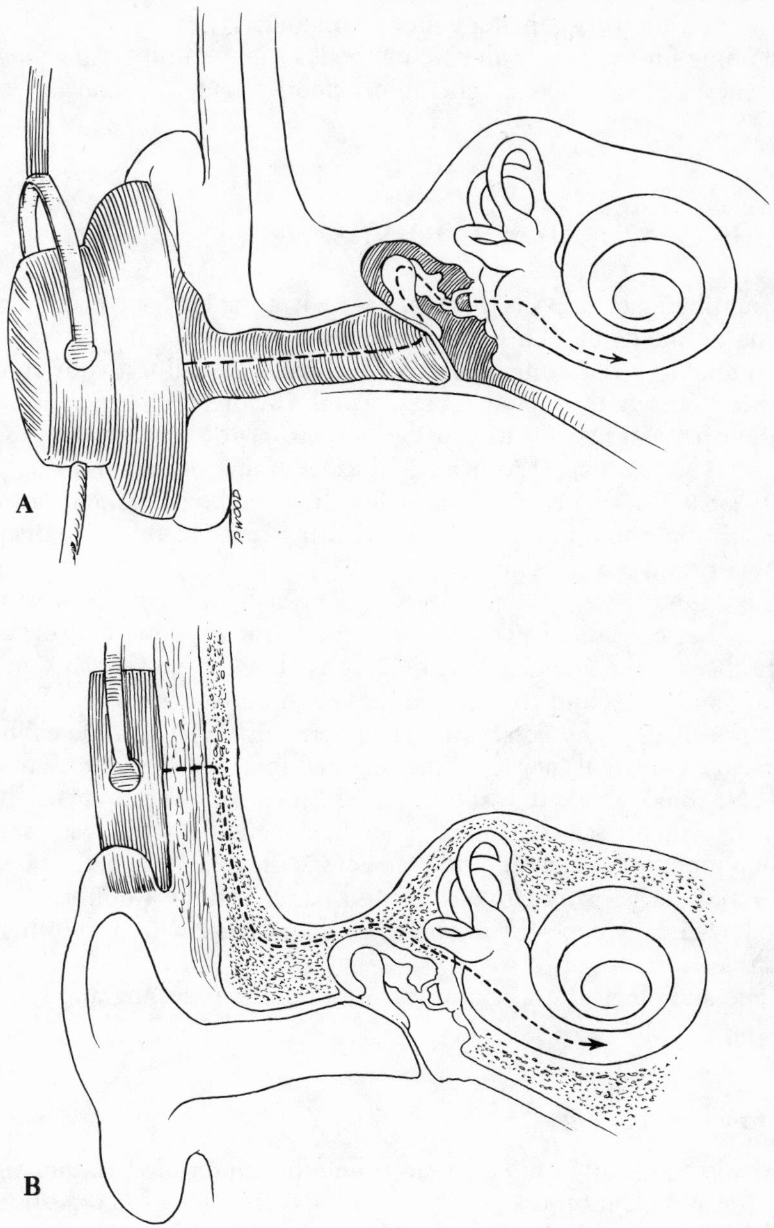

The air-conduction (A) and bone-conduction (B) pathways

a conductive hearing loss. When there is a sensorineural hearing loss, the results are usually better with air conduction.

Tuning fork tests are valuable methods for a preliminary diagnosis, but they do not yield precise information about the state of your hearing.

SEEING AN AUDIOLOGIST

If your physician suspects that you have a hearing loss, a measurement of the sensitivity of your hearing by a trained audiologist is necessary. An audiologist is a nonmedical professional who will test your ability to hear various tones and spoken words. Before testing begins, the audiologist will explain to you the purpose of the test, what types of sounds you can expect to hear, and exactly how you should respond to these tones. Many ENT specialists have audiometers and an audiologist in their offices, so that hearing tests can be conducted promptly and conveniently.

To begin the test, you are placed in a specially insulated soundproof booth that consists of two separate compartments—one for you and the other for the audiologist. The door is closed to prevent unwanted noise, and the sound level inside the booth may be anywhere from 0 to 10 decibels. (The booth and its equipment receive routine calibrations to ensure that they meet the required specifications of the American National Standards Institute [ANSI] and produce accurate results.)

Once you are seated inside the booth, the audiologist places a set of headphones over your ears and then goes to the other side of the booth. The audiologist works from a control panel behind a double-paned window directly opposite, so you can see and speak with him or her at all times.

The audiological evaluation includes pure-tone testing and speech testing.

Pure-Tone Testing

Using a specially calibrated electronic machine called an *audiometer*, the audiologist measures your hearing threshold, which means the quietest tones you can hear from low to high. The audiometer produces a series of pure tones at various high, midrange, or low frequencies and at varying levels of loudness. In a typical test, tones are presented

Masking: Not Just "White Noise"

During your audiometric tests, the audiologist may add *masking*, or the introduction of another band of sound, to the opposite ear while one ear is being tested.

Masking helps to prevent a false reading on the test. In a quiet setting, some people with a significant hearing loss in one ear may be able to pick up sounds with their better ear. This phenomenon is called *interaural attenuation*, in which the skull transfers sound over to the cochlea of the other ear. To prevent this, the audiologist puts noise, or masking, in the other ear to keep it distracted and to prevent you from hearing the transferred sound.

Masking actually mimics situations that occur to us daily. For example, it's practically impossible to carry on a conversation when you're standing a few feet from a passing train. Similarly, if you're in a crowded movie theater and people around you are talking during the film, the chatter distracts you and interferes with your ability to hear the dialogue.

Masking itself is a complex procedure. The level of masking must be constantly adjusted to match the level of the sound stimulus. Diagnostically, masking can make or break the reliability of the tests. If the right level isn't used, the results could show that you have a conductive hearing loss when in fact there is a sensorineural problem.

at frequency levels of 1,000, 2,000, 4,000, and 8,000 hertz. When you reach the lowest level at which you can hear a certain tone, the audiologist goes on to another tone. The loudness of each tone is measured in decibels, and the result is recorded on a graph—your audiogram.

As the testing proceeds and the shape of your hearing level begins to form on the graph, the audiologist may add additional frequency levels. For example, if you have normal hearing at 1,000 hertz but show an 80-decibel hearing loss at 2,000 hertz, it's important to know how well you hear at 1,500 hertz. This kind of essential information

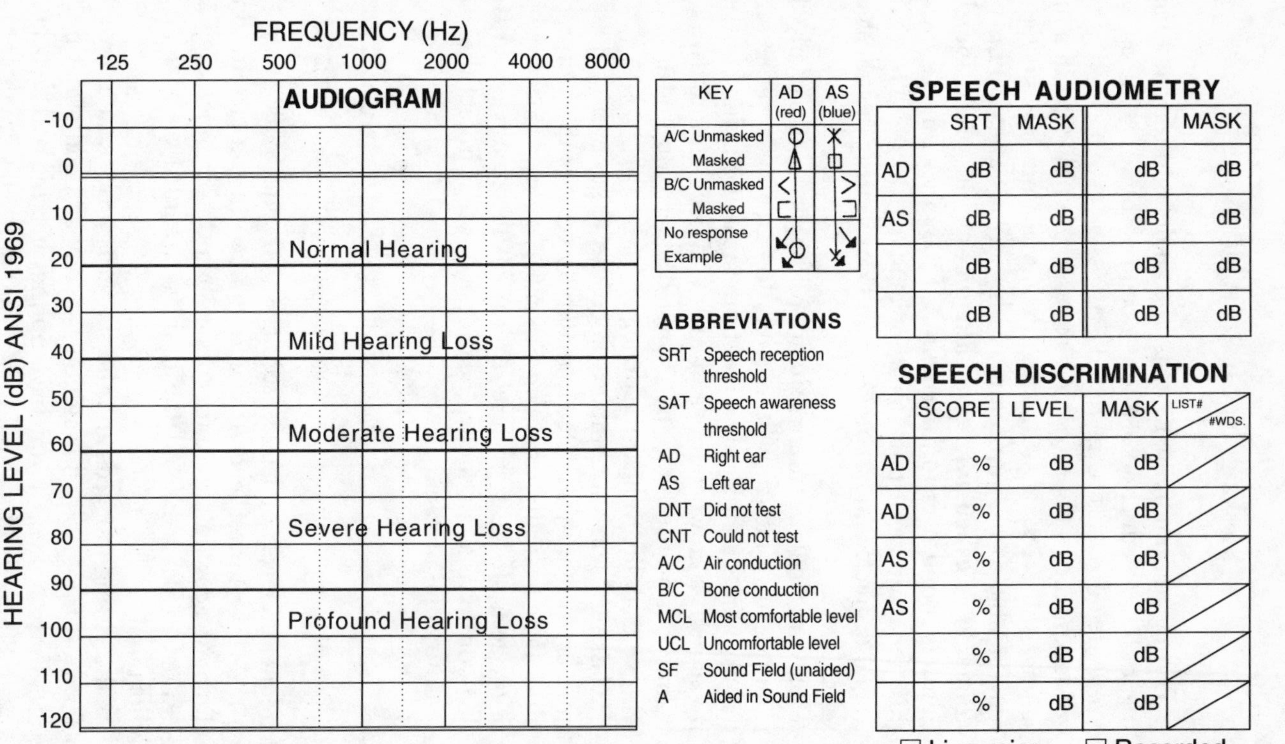

AUDIOLOGICAL EVALUATION (A)

AUDIOGRAM

KEY	AD (red)	AS (blue)
A/C Unmasked		
Masked		
B/C Unmasked	<	>
Masked		
No response Example		

ABBREVIATIONS

SRT Speech reception threshold
SAT Speech awareness threshold
AD Right ear
AS Left ear
DNT Did not test
CNT Could not test
A/C Air conduction
B/C Bone conduction
MCL Most comfortable level
UCL Uncomfortable level
SF Sound Field (unaided)
A Aided in Sound Field

SPEECH AUDIOMETRY

	SRT	MASK		MASK
AD	dB	dB	dB	dB
AS	dB	dB	dB	dB
	dB	dB	dB	dB
	dB	dB	dB	dB

SPEECH DISCRIMINATION

	SCORE	LEVEL	MASK	LIST# / #WDS.
AD	%	dB	dB	
AD	%	dB	dB	
AS	%	dB	dB	
AS	%	dB	dB	
	%	dB	dB	
	%	dB	dB	

☐ Live voice ☐ Recorded

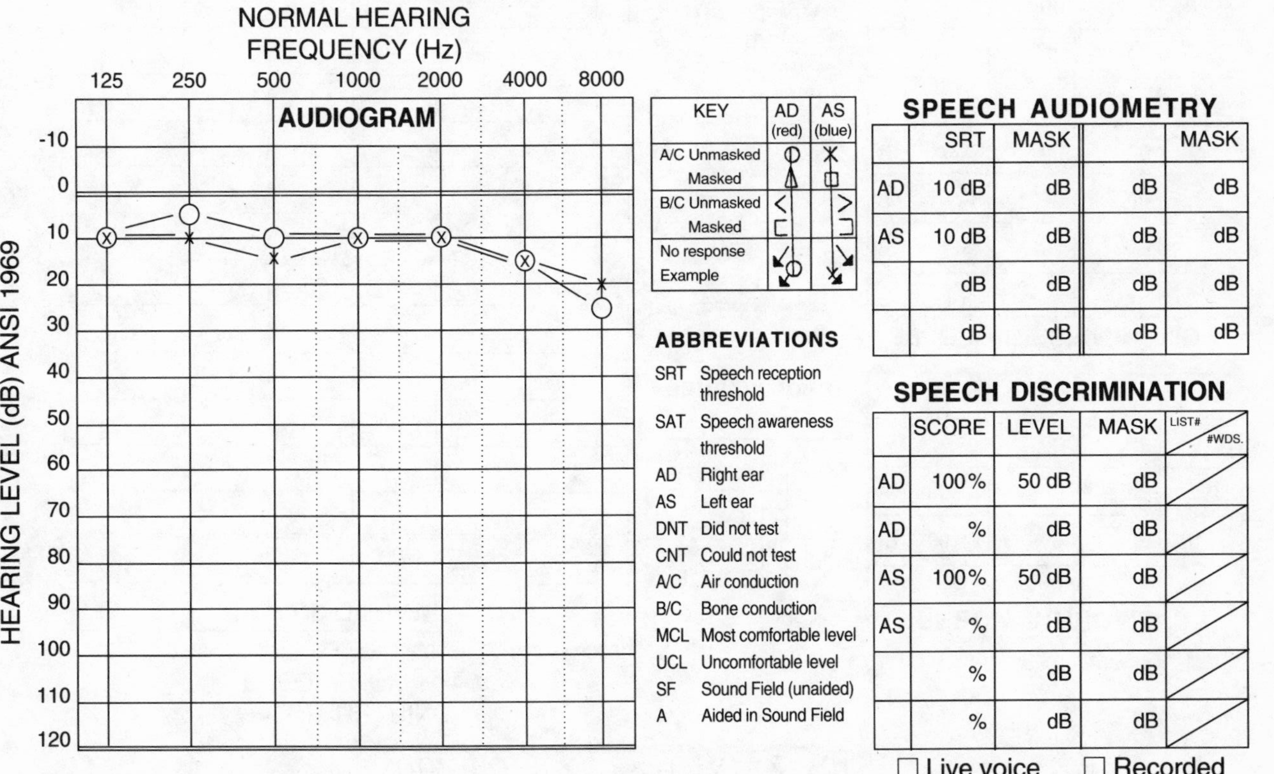

AUDIOLOGICAL EVALUATION (B)

NORMAL HEARING

FREQUENCY (Hz)

125 250 500 1000 2000 4000 8000

AUDIOGRAM

HEARING LEVEL (dB) ANSI 1969

-10 0 10 20 30 40 50 60 70 80 90 100 110 120

KEY	AD (red)	AS (blue)
A/C Unmasked	O	X
Masked	△	□
B/C Unmasked	<	>
Masked	[	]
No response	↙	↘
Example		

ABBREVIATIONS

SRT Speech reception threshold
SAT Speech awareness threshold
AD Right ear
AS Left ear
DNT Did not test
CNT Could not test
A/C Air conduction
B/C Bone conduction
MCL Most comfortable level
UCL Uncomfortable level
SF Sound Field (unaided)
A Aided in Sound Field

SPEECH AUDIOMETRY

	SRT	MASK		MASK
AD	10 dB	dB	dB	dB
AS	10 dB	dB	dB	dB
	dB	dB	dB	dB
	dB	dB	dB	dB

SPEECH DISCRIMINATION

	SCORE	LEVEL	MASK	LIST# / #WDS.
AD	100%	50 dB	dB	
AD	%	dB	dB	
AS	100%	50 dB	dB	
AS	%	dB	dB	
	%	dB	dB	
	%	dB	dB	

☐ Live voice ☐ Recorded

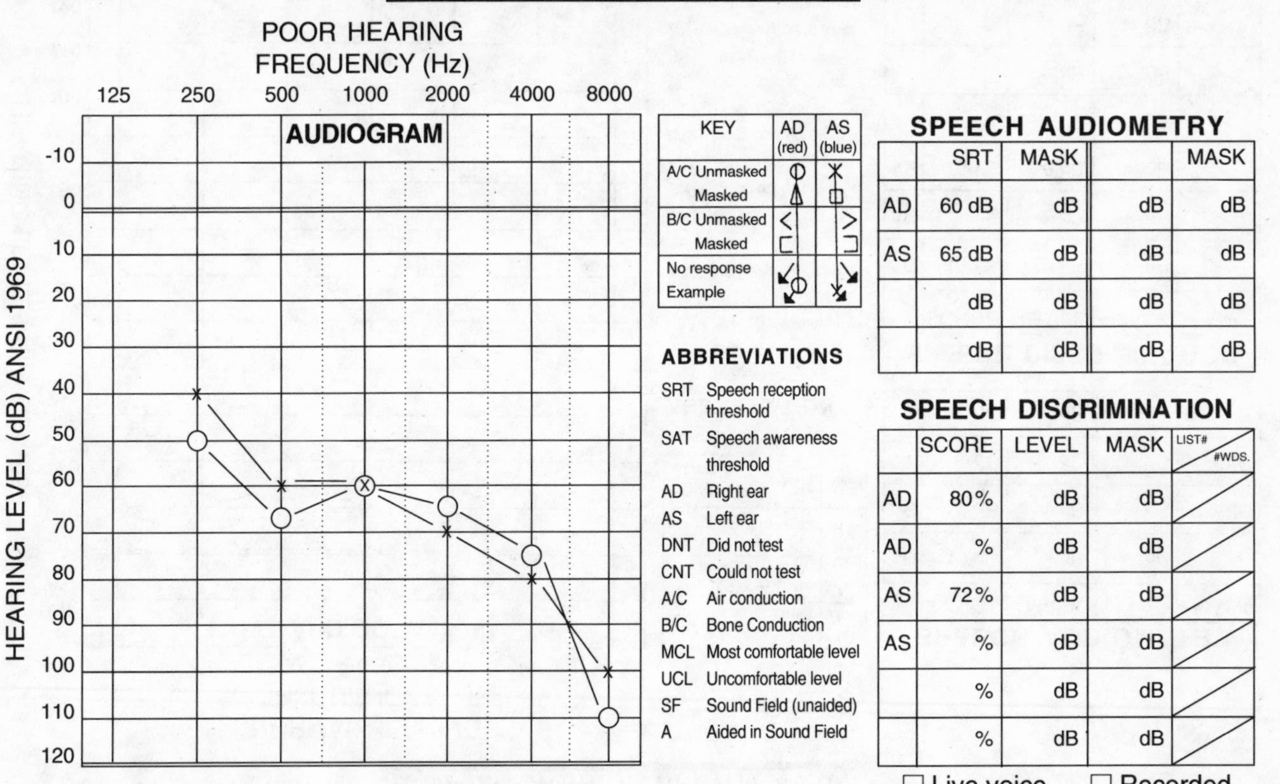

AUDIOLOGICAL EVALUATION (C)

POOR HEARING

KEY	AD (red)	AS (blue)
A/C Unmasked	○	X
Masked	△	□
B/C Unmasked	<	>
Masked	[	]
No response Example	↙○	↘X

ABBREVIATIONS

- SRT Speech reception threshold
- SAT Speech awareness threshold
- AD Right ear
- AS Left ear
- DNT Did not test
- CNT Could not test
- A/C Air conduction
- B/C Bone Conduction
- MCL Most comfortable level
- UCL Uncomfortable level
- SF Sound Field (unaided)
- A Aided in Sound Field

SPEECH AUDIOMETRY

	SRT	MASK		MASK
AD	60 dB	dB	dB	dB
AS	65 dB	dB	dB	dB
	dB	dB	dB	dB
	dB	dB	dB	dB

SPEECH DISCRIMINATION

	SCORE	LEVEL	MASK	LIST# / #WDS.
AD	80%	dB	dB	
AD	%	dB	dB	
AS	72%	dB	dB	
AS	%	dB	dB	
	%	dB	dB	
	%	dB	dB	

☐ Live voice ☐ Recorded

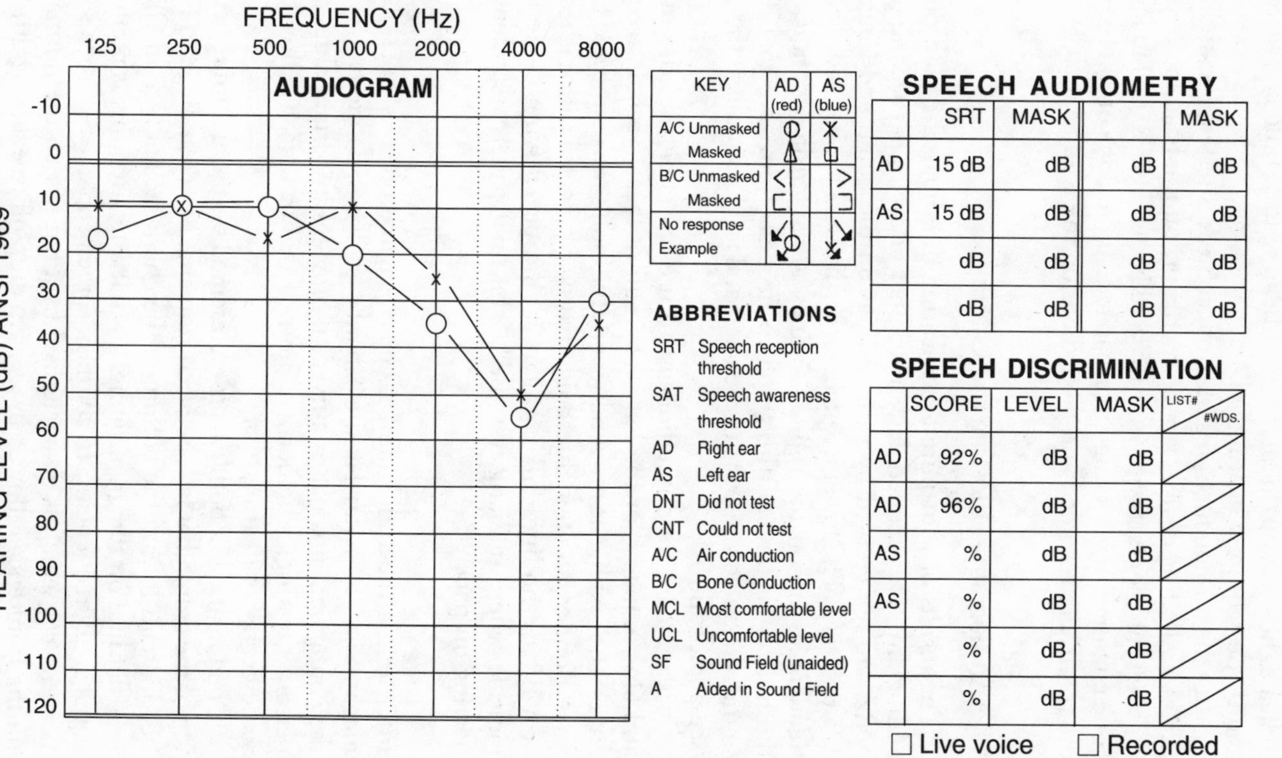
AUDIOLOGICAL EVALUATION (D)
NOISE NOTCH
FREQUENCY (Hz)
125 250 500 1000 2000 4000 8000
AUDIOGRAM
HEARING LEVEL (dB) ANSI 1969
-10 0 10 20 30 40 50 60 70 80 90 100 110 120
KEY | AD (red) | AS (blue)
A/C Unmasked
Masked
B/C Unmasked
Masked
No response
Example
ABBREVIATIONS
SRT Speech reception threshold
SAT Speech awareness threshold
AD Right ear
AS Left ear
DNT Did not test
CNT Could not test
A/C Air conduction
B/C Bone Conduction
MCL Most comfortable level
UCL Uncomfortable level
SF Sound Field (unaided)
A Aided in Sound Field
SPEECH AUDIOMETRY
SRT | MASK | | MASK
AD | 15 dB | dB | dB | dB
AS | 15 dB | dB | dB | dB
dB | dB | dB | dB
dB | dB | dB | dB
SPEECH DISCRIMINATION
SCORE | LEVEL | MASK | LIST# #WDS.
AD | 92% | dB | dB
AD | 96% | dB | dB
AS | % | dB | dB
AS | % | dB | dB
% | dB | dB
% | dB | dB
Live voice
Recorded

indicates how your particular type of hearing loss could best be treated, and if you require a hearing aid.

After the air-conduction ability of each ear is tested, the audiologist places a vibrating device, a bone oscillator, on the headphones so that it comes into contact with your mastoid bone. This is used to test your bone conduction. Once again, separate tests are done on each ear, and the results are recorded and plotted out on the audiogram.

The Audiogram—Plotting the Graph

The results of your pure-tone hearing thresholds are placed on the audiogram. The frequencies, or number of cycles per second (cps) or hertz, are represented by vertical lines on the graph and range from 125 to 8,000. The lower frequencies are listed at the left and the higher frequencies are on the right. Loudness, or intensity, is indicated on the horizontal lines of the graph in decibels from zero to 120. Soft sounds are noted at the top of the chart and louder sounds at the bottom (see audiogram A).

It is standard for an audiologist to use red circles for the right ear and blue X marks for the left. When all of these symbols are plotted out on the graph, the air conduction thresholds are connected by solid lines. Bone conduction thresholds may be connected with dashed lines, or will have no lines linking them at all. Special symbols are used to indicate where masking was used. The final pattern represents your hearing on paper.

Interpreting the audiogram. The configuration, or shape, of an audiogram is as individual as the patient—each one is different. Whether the configuration is flat or curved, it provides important clues about a person's hearing, whether it is normal or not, and whether there is some degree of hearing loss.

Good hearing in both ears is represented by a straight line across the top of the graph that falls between zero and 20 (see audiogram B). Poor hearing falls toward the bottom of the chart (see audiogram C).

A flat line on the graph indicates that a hearing loss is pretty much equal at all frequencies. In contrast, some people may have a so-called *noise notch*, which is characterized by a flat line in the normal range on the front end, followed by a sharp drop-off (see audiogram D).

Early damage to hearing from exposure to excessive noise typically shows up in audiological testing as a lowered sensitivity to sounds in the 4,000-hertz range. With continued exposure to such noise, hearing progressively diminishes in both the higher and lower frequencies. Eventually, the audiogram begins to resemble that of a person with presbycusis, or age-related hearing loss.

A different kind of notch, called a *Carhart notch*, often appears on the audiogram of a person with otosclerosis. In this middle-ear disorder, the foot plate of the tiny stapes bone becomes fixated in the oval window leading to the inner ear (see chapter 2).

To further test your hearing, the audiologist administers a speech test.

SPEECH TESTING

When you listen to someone talking, you must hear it *and* understand what you are hearing. Two tests measure your speech reception threshold and your ability to discriminate words.

Speech Reception Threshold

The minimum level at which you can identify words used in simple speech is your *speech reception threshold (SRT)*. The purpose of the SRT is not to determine the level at which you can just barely detect the presence of speech, but to find the level at which you can identify words and repeat 50 percent of them correctly.

In this test, the audiologist states a familiar word or plays a tape of prerecorded words and asks you to repeat each one. The words used are called spondees, two-syllable words that have an equal stress on each syllable. When testing begins, the words come into the soundproof booth at a level that you can easily hear. For example, the tester may say "baseball" and you repeat "baseball." Next may come the word "hot dog" and you repeat it. Then "cupcake," and so on down the list of words.

Speech Discrimination

Testing your ability to understand words is performed at a level that is well above your hearing threshold. The words are loud enough to be easily heard, but not uncomfortably so.

Degrees of Hearing Loss

When testing is completed and the results of your audiogram have been plotted, your hearing level is classified by the degree of impairment as measured against a standardized chart. The degrees of hearing loss range from mild to severe:

0–20 decibels	Normal hearing
20–45 decibels	Mild hearing loss
45–60 decibels	Moderate hearing loss
60–75 decibels	Moderately severe hearing loss
75–90 decibels	Severe hearing loss
90 and above	Profound hearing loss

The words used in discrimination testing contain only one syllable. They might include familiar words such as *our*, *jar*, and *this*. These words come from specially designed lists of phonetically balanced words that have a similar distribution of vowels and consonants as those occurring in everyday speech. The audiologist may present these words to you in his or her own voice or in a prerecorded format.

Your score is determined by the percentage of words that you repeat correctly. If you've repeated all of the words correctly, your score is 100 percent. A speech discrimination score that ranges between 90 and 100 percent is considered normal.

Scoring high on a discrimination test does not mean that your hearing is good. But when your discrimination score is considered along with the first part of speech testing—your ability to hear speech normally—it helps the audiologist determine whether you could benefit from some kind of assistive listening device.

Someone who has normal speech discrimination, but whose hearing level is borderline, may get excellent results with a hearing aid. It amplifies words so they can be understood clearly. But a person with poor discrimination whose hearing falls within the normal range may not do as well with a hearing aid and may need only to learn special listening techniques (see chapter 9).

Making the Diagnosis

The audiogram and the speech tests both provide valuable information, but this is not a diagnosis. When the results of your audiological workup are ready, they are given to your physician, who then makes a diagnosis based on the tests in combination with your medical history and the findings from your physical examination.

If further medical treatment is necessary, your doctor will explain the problem to you and recommend possible solutions. Often, the audiologist's tests point to the need for an assistive listening device or instruction in speechreading. However, in the case of a woman with a Carhart notch on her audiogram (see page 65) and a history of early hearing loss among women in her family, surgical treatment may be recommended to correct the problem. When a hearing aid is necessary, the audiologist may be able to provide one or recommend another qualified professional who is licensed to dispense these products.

OTHER HEARING TESTS

The audiologist can obtain additional information about middle-ear functioning by using other instruments and tests. The most common of these tests is *tympanometry*, which measures the movement of the eardrum in response to changes in air pressure.

The patient sits quietly while an earplug is placed first in one ear and then in the other. Through a tube attached to the plug, the audiologist introduces negative and positive pressure into the ear canal.

The tympanometer automatically records the maximum movement of the eardrum at different pressure levels and produces a graph that indicates where the most motion occurred. If there is no eardrum motion, it may indicate the presence of fluid in the middle ear. When the highest level of eardrum motion registers as a negative number, it may indicate that the eustachian tube (the drainage tube for the ear) is not opening and closing normally.

Tympanometry is especially useful for young children and those who, because of illness or injury, have difficulty responding to test directions. Because fluid in the middle ear is common among children, many pediatricians have a tympanometer in their offices to identify and treat youngsters with this problem.

Tympanometry is not a 100 percent accurate test, however. For this reason, it's usually used in conjunction with a physical examination to diagnose the presence of fluid in the middle ear.

Evoked Response Audiometry

Similar to the electroencephalogram that a neurologist uses to measure the electrical activity of brain waves, evoked response audiometry (ERA) follows sound as it goes from the inner ear through the auditory nerve and on to the brain.

ERA testing is very useful for two major diagnostic problems. It can be used to measure the threshold, or lowest level of hearing, in people who can't or won't offer accurate responses to standard hearing testing—newborns, small children, even litigants in legal cases. ERA also can help reveal hearing problems that are not necessarily located in the ears. For example, a tumor may be pressing on the nerve that allows sound conduction. Diseases like multiple sclerosis (MS) may also cause

Infants at High Risk of Hearing Loss

A joint policy statement on infant hearing was issued in 1990 by the American Speech-Language-Hearing Association, the American Academy of Otolaryngology, the American Academy of Pediatrics, and the Council for Education of the Deaf.

These recommendations expand the list of previously used criteria for identifying newborns at high risk of hearing loss. The criteria include:

- family history of hearing loss
- congenital infection
- malformations of the ear
- low birthweight
- hyperbilirubinemia
- bacterial meningitis
- severe asphyxia
- more than 10 days on a mechanical ventilator
- use of medications that are toxic to the ear
- physical signs associated with a genetic syndrome, such as Waardenburg's syndrome

Some of the same criteria apply to children from four weeks to two years of age, including bacterial meningitis. Additional criteria for this older age group include:

- concern by the parent or caregiver regarding delays in the child's hearing, speech, or language and/or development
- traumatic injury to the head
- degenerative disorders of the nervous system
- childhood infectious diseases, such as mumps and measles

Once hearing loss has been established, the child should undergo an evaluation by a hearing specialist and have an audiological workup. When a child is hearing-impaired, a speech-language pathologist or similar professional can develop a program and recommend communication devices to assist the child in language and communication development.

Of course, the above criteria do not identify all children with hearing loss, only those who are at high risk. To identify all children with hearing problems, it would be necessary to screen every child.

abnormal sound conduction. In MS, the nerve activity is short-circuited when the myelin insulation that covers the spinal nerves deteriorates.

First, sticky pads that contain electrodes are placed on the head. These electrodes are hooked up to a computer. Repetitive clicks or tones are then played into the ear through an earphone. As the computer registers and records the brain's response, the hearing information is electronically extracted from other electrical activity that normally occurs in the brain stem.

ERA is also known as brain-stem evoked response audiometry (BER), auditory evoked response (AER), or auditory brain-stem response (ABR).

Computerized Tomography and Magnetic Resonance Imaging

The specialist may order additional tests if standard tests or evoked response audiometry testing is abnormal or does not offer conclusive information, or if the patient's medical history does not offer enough clues to explain the cause of the hearing loss.

Computed tomography (CT) or magnetic resonance imaging (MRI) is especially valuable in detecting very small growths, demyelinating disease, and any vascular abnormalities in the brain.

HEARING LOSS IN CHILDREN

Beginning at birth, a child learns how to communicate by listening, imitating noises, responding to sound, gesturing, and learning how to use language. After associating different sounds with their meanings, the child begins to understand what people are saying, and develops a sense of how to use language. But in order to use language, a child must first be able to hear.

Unfortunately, hearing loss in children often goes unrecognized until a parent or teacher notices that the youngster seems to lag behind other children in the same age group. A child may be too young to express or even understand that something is wrong, and it may not be until a delay in speech and language development becomes apparent that a hearing loss is detected.

Early identification of hearing problems is essential for a child to develop normal language and social skills. For this reason, children should have their hearing screened routinely, beginning at birth.

Normal Behavior and Hearing Response in a Child

The acquisition of motor skills, social interaction, and language are among the important milestones that mark the stages of a child's development. Of course, not every child develops at the same rate. Just as one child may begin to walk at nine months, another may not take that first step until many months later. And so it is with speech and language skills: The rates at which children acquire language vary widely.

It's important to follow your child's progress at each stage of development and to have some knowledge of what to expect. In this way many alert parents and teachers have identified a hearing problem in a child early, when effective remedial steps could be taken.

A child's ability to hear is reflected in certain forms of behavior at various age levels:

Age	Response to Sound
Birth to 3 months	Startled by loud sounds. Is soothed or quieted from crying by mother's voice.
3–6 months	Turns eyes or head to locate the source of sound. Responds to mother's voice. Enjoys sound-making toys, such as rattles. Copies some sounds, such as "ba-ba," "da-da," "ma-ma."
6–10 months	Responds to own name, a ringing telephone, voices. Understands "no," "bye-bye."
10–15 months	When asked to identify a familiar person or object, can point to it. Imitates simple words and sounds.
15–18 months	Follows simple spoken directions. Uses a handful of real "first words." Shows a steady growth in speech and language skills.
2 years	Enjoys listening and being read to. Refers to self by name. Makes incomplete or grammatically incomplete sentences: "Milk all gone."
2½ years	Recites or sings short songs and enjoys listening to music. Reacts appropriately to heard sounds without having any visual cues, such as the doorbell or a ringing telephone.
3 years	Uses complete sentences some of the time. Understands and uses "go" and "me."

Children of school age who may have some degree of hearing loss often have certain characteristic behaviors, including:

- Failing to pay attention when spoken to casually
- Often asking a person who is speaking to repeat words or sentences
- Giving wrong or inappropriate answers to simple questions

- "Hearing" better when watching the face of the speaker
- Functioning below ability at school
- Ignoring what a parent or teacher says, and behavior becomes a problem
- Developing frequent earaches, colds, and upper respiratory infections, and may suffer from hayfever
- Speech articulation (pronunciation) is not clear
- Withdrawing from children of similar age or from classmates

If your child doesn't respond to sound as suggested here, or if he or she demonstrates the behavior listed above, consult your pediatrician.

Audiology Testing in Children

To test an infant's or a child's hearing, the audiologist uses a variety of different techniques. These include behavioral observation, visual reinforcement, play audiometry, and evoked response audiometry.

The tests chosen are based on a child's age:

Birth to six months. If there is a question about a baby's ability to hear, the infant will be referred to a specialist who conducts evoked response audiometry (ERA). Because infants can't stay still for a long period of time, and because their behavioral responses aren't very well developed, ERA offers an objective way to explore an infant's sense of hearing.

Six to twelve months. A technique known as *behavioral observation audiometry* is helpful at this stage. The baby sits on the mother's lap at an equal distance between two speakers. The audiologist then presents a variety of sound stimuli at different volume levels while closely observing any changes in the child's behavior.

Among the clues the audiologist looks for are whether the child shows a startle reaction to any of the sounds or becomes quieter. Any changes in breathing or facial expression, such as widening of the eyes, also are noted.

12 to 18 months. For this age group, behavior observation is usually combined with *visual reinforcement audiometry*.

The basic technique in visual reinforcement testing is similar to Pavlovian conditioning, in which the subject being tested becomes conditioned to receiving a reward for acting or answering correctly. In this case, the audiologist "conditions" the child to locate a sound and turn toward its source. When the child is successful, the visual reinforcement or reward is a stimulus, such as a puppet that lights up or a toy that bursts into animated activity.

To condition the child, the audiologist pairs the sound with the visual reinforcement at a volume level that the child can hear. Once the child is conditioned, testing begins.

20 months and older. Beginning at this age, an audiologist can make use of *play audiometry*, in which the child is tested by means of various kinds of play activities.

Earphones are placed on the child, and the audiologist asks him or her to play certain games, such as putting rings on a stick, dropping blocks in a bucket, or pointing to a picture. Using pure-tone stimuli at various low, midrange, and high frequencies, the audiologist tests the child's hearing threshold. During the conditioning period, the child is allowed to play the game only when a sound stimulus occurs: He or she can place a ring on the stick only after hearing a tone through the earphones.

During pure-tone testing, the audiologist checks air conduction as well as bone conduction. Adult testing techniques can be used also, depending on the child's mental and emotional development, hearing level, and ability to understand and follow directions.

Because children tire easily and may not be able to focus their attention for very long, an audiological evaluation of a young child may require more than one session in order to achieve a complete audiogram.

Tympanometry tests are also conducted in young children. The results of these tests are considered along with the audiogram, the child's history, and physical examination when the physician makes a diagnosis.

Treating the Hearing-Impaired Child

When a child is diagnosed as having a hearing loss, immediate treatment is necessary. In some cases an otolaryngologist may be able to medically treat the cause of the problem. For example, if there is fluid behind the eardrum, medications or surgery may be recommended. If the hearing loss is not correctable, the treatment depends upon the degree of loss.

Coping with the Diagnosis

Finding out that your child has a moderate or a severe hearing loss is devastating. You may go through a process of mourning as you try to cope with the realization that your child may never hear normally. Eventually, though, you will realize that you must play the central role in arranging for treatment and therapy so your child can develop communication skills.

Of course, professionals are available to offer counseling and support. A speech-language pathologist can evaluate your child's special learning needs and prescribe the proper therapy. A speech instructor can teach the child the fundamentals of speech and language. And special schools are available for children with severe hearing loss.

But these experts cannot reverse the hearing loss or take full responsibility for helping your child. It takes a great deal of time, patience, effort, and support for a severely hearing-impaired child to first learn language and speech skills. If you consider yourself a part of the team, you can learn how to work with the experts and encourage your child to adjust to his or her hearing impairment. You can make all the difference in whether or not your child does well in school and in society.

(For more information on coping with a hearing loss, see chapter 9.)

Some children require nothing more than preferential seating in school; others may need a hearing aid. Speech therapy is usually recommended for most hearing-impaired children, however. It is also critical that children with hearing loss are regularly seen by a specialist during childhood and throughout their teen years, or until their problem is corrected.

A child who is able to fully hear from one ear can be expected to develop and use language in a normal manner, although he or she will miss words that are spoken near the impaired ear. A youngster with a mild conductive hearing loss in both ears may have difficulty hearing speech from a distance. No special treatment is usually necessary for these children, other than seating them in the front of the classroom so they can hear the teacher.

When the diagnosis is a severe sensorineural hearing loss, the child will require a great deal of instruction in speech and language development. If he or she has even a small amount of hearing, amplification with a hearing aid may be beneficial. Children who are found to be completely deaf, or who become deaf, face a special set of problems and solutions (see chapter 9).

TESTING HEARING AT SCHOOL AND ON THE JOB

Schoolchildren and industrial workers are often required to take screening tests for their hearing. These tests use specialized equipment that can help identify a potential hearing problem.

Screenings in Schools

Today, most school districts conduct hearing tests of all their pupils. Although testing may not be performed annually in every state, it usually is conducted once every two or three years, and when a new student transfers into a district.

Hearing tests in schools usually consist of air conduction studies, which are the first part of pure-tone testing. The screenings may be administered in the school nurse's office or in mobile testing units that travel to each school.

If a child fails a test and then does equally poorly when retested, the parents are alerted and advised that a medical evaluation is necessary. For some children, the diagnosis may be a hearing problem, while for others there also may be an underlying learning disability.

In recent years, some states have begun adding tympanometry to the standard regimen of school hearing tests.

Screenings in Industry

Audiometric screening is conducted by many industries—for new workers as a prerequisite of employment and also for workers who are exposed to high levels of noise on the job.

Identification audiometry is administered to new employees before they begin work with a new employer. The result of this screening is called a "reference audiogram" because the company will refer to it for comparison purposes as future audiograms are taken.

When an incoming employee is tested and found to have especially sensitive ears, the company is alerted that this worker could suffer a hearing loss if assigned to a noisy work area. A firm that ignores such a finding and places this worker in a noisy location runs the risk years later of receiving a worker's compensation claim for hearing loss.

Monitoring audiometry is used to detect any changes in hearing that may have occurred *after* the preemployment screening test. When monitoring audiometry shows any significant difference from the reference audiogram, the worker should receive a full medical evaluation by a hearing specialist and a hearing evaluation by an audiologist.

Both identification and monitoring audiometry are usually administered to workers in an automated format known as a *sweep check test*. This type of screening can be given to several people at one time. The audiologist or specially trained technician who conducts the testing instructs the test takers in what to expect and how to respond to what they hear.

4

Selecting, Buying, and Using a Hearing Aid

In ancient times, people placed a cupped hand behind the ear in order to hear more effectively. Much later, the hard-of-hearing used mechanical ear trumpets, and still later, clumsy hearing devices that were the precursors of today's modern hearing aids.

However crude the early hearing instruments, their purpose was the same as that of modern aids: to amplify sound. The acoustic devices of previous centuries were largely ineffective, though, because their usefulness was limited to gathering and directing sound waves to the ear, thereby increasing the intensity of sound by only a few decibels.

Today, state-of-the-art hearing aids can increase sound intensity by as much as 60 to 70 decibels. Technological advances also now permit the installation of many built-in options, such as a noise-suppression switch and circuitry that amplifies soft-to-medium sounds without also amplifying louder noises.

Such innovation has produced several different styles and types of hearing aids. After former president Ronald Reagan appeared in public wearing a hearing aid in 1983, most Americans became familiar with in-the-canal aids. Depending on an individual's needs, other styles—such as those worn behind the ear—may be more desirable or effective, however.

BEFORE YOU BUY A HEARING AID

It has been estimated that each year countless Americans buy hearing aids that prove to be of little value. Mail-order houses, door-to-door salespeople, and companies that directly advertise their hearing aids to consumers through magazines and on TV make a number of claims about their products but don't always deliver what they promise.

One industry survey found that 40 percent of people who bought hearing aids were less than fully satisfied with the experience, and consumer complaints to state licensing boards show some of the reasons. An unscrupulous hearing-aid dealer may try to sell you the hearing aid with the largest profit margin, rather than the one best suited to your needs. Dealers have even fitted people with hearing aids they didn't need at all; in one reported case, a hearing aid was sold to someone whose only problem was wax in his ears. Many people find they have difficulty getting a hearing aid adjusted or replaced, or the cost refunded, when the aid doesn't work as promised.

Of course, newcomers to hearing aids have certain expectations that may or may not be fulfilled. Unlike buying a pair of eyeglasses and readily adapting to the new, sharper images they provide, using a hearing aid successfully is more of an acquired skill.

So it's no wonder that hearing aids have earned a bad reputation, especially among those who bought a low-quality or poor-fitting instrument. Unfortunately, many of these disgruntled consumers not only give up on hearing aids but also tell others that hearing aids are not worth the expense.

To avoid disappointment and dissatisfaction, anyone who is considering the purchase of a hearing aid is advised to first consult with an otologist or otolaryngologist, who can guide them to a qualified audiologist. If it is determined, after a series of tests, that a hearing aid can help you, the audiologist can also recommend the best style and type of device for your particular level of hearing loss.

The actual purchase of a hearing aid may be from an audiologist who is specially trained to dispense hearing aids, or from a qualified dealer. (*Note:* Some audiologists sell hearing aids and are in competition with dealers. For this reason, when the term *dispenser* is used in these pages, it applies to both of these providers.) In either case, you are not just buying a device for your personal use. You are actually contracting with the dispenser for an entire package of services, including routine servicing of your hearing aid as well as training in how to operate it effectively.

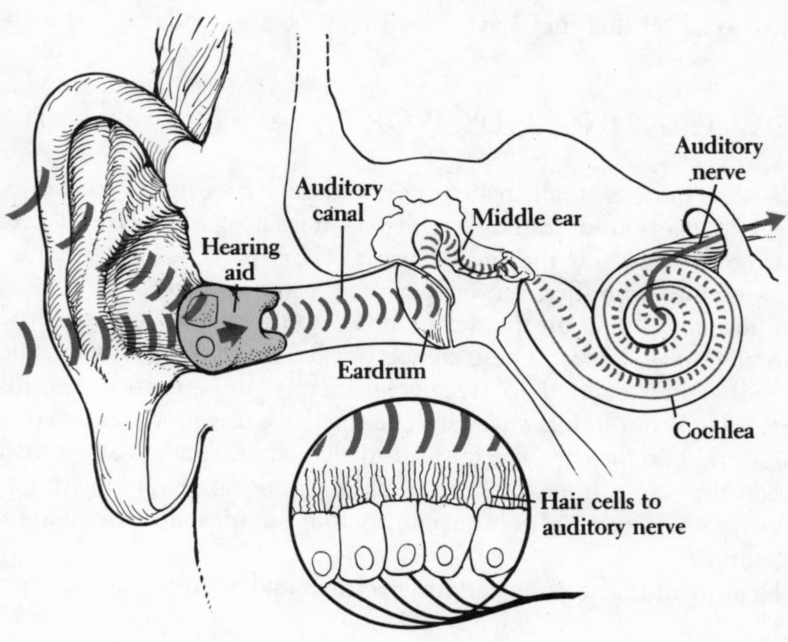

Sound enters the ear as vibrations of the air. In a hearing aid, these vibrations are converted to an electrical signal (arrow), which can be amplified. The hearing aid then emits the amplified sound waves, which are conveyed by way of the bones in the middle ear to the cochlea. In the cochlea, hair cells (shown magnified in the circle) convert these vibrations to nerve signals, which travel through the auditory nerve to the brain.

Many aspects need to be considered when you buy a hearing aid. Practical considerations such as style, type, and cost are important, but your own feelings about wearing a hearing device are even more vital. Not surprisingly, those who report poor results with a hearing aid often refuse to admit that they have a hearing problem at all.

HOW HEARING AIDS WORK

A hearing aid is a small, battery-powered device worn in, on, or near the ear that amplifies sounds for the person wearing it. Practically every hearing aid contains the same basic working parts, which include a microphone, amplifier, receiver, batteries, and earpiece.

The microphone on the device picks up the sound and converts it into electrical signals. These signals are fed into an amplifier, which increases their strength. A receiver converts the amplified electrical signals back into sound waves and, acting like a tiny loudspeaker, sends the sound into the ear. The custom-made earpiece, called an *earmold*, directs the sound from the hearing aid into the ear. Every hearing aid comes with an external volume control that can make the sound louder or softer.

Hearing aids also have certain electrical and acoustical characteristics.

Common Characteristics of Hearing Aids

The audiologist or hearing aid dealer may use certain technical terms when fitting you with a hearing aid. These terms apply to such properties as gain, output, frequency response, and frequency range.

Gain. This refers to the hearing aid's power, or ability to amplify sound. Gain is the number of decibels that a hearing aid can add to sound.

Output. The loudest sound that a hearing aid can produce, no matter how loud the incoming sound, is its output (also called maximum power output). This characteristic is designed to protect the ears of a hearing aid wearer from uncomfortably loud or damaging sounds.

Frequency response. The frequency response is the gain that a hearing aid has across different frequencies.

Frequency range. How much the instrument can amplify in both the high and low frequencies is its frequency range. Depending on the hearing aid, sound amplification can be effective from the low frequencies—beginning at 500 cycles per second—up to 3,000 cycles at the higher end of the range.

The frequencies that occur in speech—especially the consonant sounds that are important in understanding words—begin at a frequency range of about 2,000 and can go as high as 6,000 to 8,000 hertz. Spoken consonants don't stay in one particular pitch or frequency but are spread across a range of frequencies.

Engineers have not yet been able to design a hearing aid that effectively amplifies at 4,000 cycles and above.

BENEFITS AND LIMITATIONS OF HEARING AIDS

A hearing aid can be enormously helpful if you suffer from hearing loss—as long as you remain aware of its limitations. A hearing aid is not a "new" ear. It won't restore your hearing, but it *can* make a major difference in helping you communicate with others.

Learning how to use a hearing aid effectively takes a little time, but most satisfied users say it is a skill worth mastering. Yet, there are many myths surrounding hearing aids.

What a Hearing Aid Can Do

Hearing aids are worn for the amplification that these devices can produce. A hearing aid can make the sounds of speech comfortably louder for listening and help you to better understand conversation. As a side benefit, other people usually make an effort to speak more clearly when they notice that you are wearing a hearing aid.

Depending on the degree of your hearing loss, a hearing aid can increase your environmental awareness of important sounds, such as doors opening, horns honking, telephones ringing, and visitors knocking at the door.

What a Hearing Aid Cannot Do

Although a hearing aid makes sounds louder, it doesn't necessarily mean that the *clarity* of what you hear is automatically improved.

Depending on the nature of your hearing loss and your distance from a speaker, you may not understand every spoken word. Because a hearing aid picks up more sounds, however, it enables you to use these sounds and any visual cues to help fill in the blanks.

Another major limitation of hearing aids is that they don't just amplify what you *want* to hear. Instead, they tend to amplify both the signal you're trying to hear as well as other noises around you. These include common noises like running water, the motors of appliances, and even the sounds that your jaw and mouth make as you chew your food.

A hearing aid cannot restore sound quality to its natural state. Just as a concert heard on the radio sounds different from a live performance, the electrical reception will change the quality of what you hear. As a result, sound received through a hearing aid tends to be perceived as one step removed, or slightly artificial.

Researchers and engineers are constantly working to overcome many of these limitations. In fact, the new generation of hearing aids does much more than just make a sound louder; the more sophisticated units can be adjusted to compensate for the natural patterns of hearing loss. This kind of technological advance helps to eliminate the most common complaint about hearing aids—that they duplicate background noises as well as speech.

Depending on the degree—or amount—of your hearing loss, certain types of hearing aids may better meet your particular needs. Another important consideration is the *configuration*, or shape, of your hearing loss. This aspect influences your ability to understand all of the sounds that occur in speech.

Configuration of Hearing Loss

The actual shape of your hearing, or its configuration on an audiogram, is a reflection of where your hearing loss occurs across the normal range of frequencies.

Sometimes, hearing loss occurs in a recognizable shape on the graph. A *saucer-shaped* hearing loss is characterized by its slightly curved slope on an audiogram—a shape that indicates that hearing is better on the lower and higher ends of the frequency range than in the middle. A *precipitous* hearing loss resembles a ski slope. In this case, hearing is nearly normal at the lower frequencies, but falls dramatically beginning in the midrange frequencies.

Age-related hearing loss, or presbycusis, can fall into a fairly predictable configuration, although the degree of impairment is different for each person. With aging, hearing loss seems to occur first in the higher frequencies, only gradually spreading into the lower frequencies later on.

The pattern of hearing loss may occasionally take a certain shape, but more often it does not. When a hearing aid is appropriate, it must be carefully designed to match the configuration and degree of each person's particular pattern of loss.

Selecting a hearing aid is a highly personal choice. Many other variables enter the picture, including one's age, social and professional demands, and individual listening needs.

TYPES OF HEARING AIDS

In the not-too-distant past, hearing aids were all alike—there was only one model. Today new developments in technology have expanded the selection and given people a choice of conventional, digitally controlled, or programmable hearing aids.

Conventional Hearing Aids

A conventional, or analog, hearing aid is basically an amplifier. Analog technology has been used to transmit television broadcasts for decades. In television, the pictures received on the screen are electrical representations of the original images that were sent out. Similarly, when a sound impulse enters a hearing aid, the aid amplifies the analog signal, which is actually an imitation of the original acoustic energy pattern.

A conventional hearing aid amplifies across a certain frequency range. The range itself is selected by an audiologist and is based on your particular needs. Because the aid amplifies an entire spectrum of sound—as opposed to just what you want to hear—selective amplification is difficult because the device picks up environmental noises as well.

It is possible to have a special feature built into a conventional hearing aid that adjusts the tone of the amplification in both the lower and higher frequencies. Special circuitry that reduces background noise or filters out some of the environmental din can also be requested for a conventional model. A dispenser can make any necessary changes or adjustments of certain settings right in the office.

Advantages. A conventional hearing aid, with an available menu of special options, is usually recommended for first-time hearing aid users. As long as it has been properly fitted, this type of traditional hearing device usually can improve most hearing problems.

A conventional hearing aid is lower in cost, too. The price increases significantly, however, depending on the circuitry or other options selected.

Disadvantages. As mentioned previously, this type of hearing aid tends to make *all* sounds louder—not just the ones you want to hear. Also, the clarity of sound may not be ideal.

Digitally Controlled Hearing Aids

The digital technology that has been successfully applied to musical recordings and to high-definition television has been found to offer great promise to hearing aid wearers as well.

The term *digital* comes from computers, where it refers to the numerical values that are assigned to certain functions within the computer's electronic memory. In its application to hearing, this technology is being used to control and modify sound, from when it first enters the microphone to when it leaves the receiver to enter your ear.

When musical recordings are digitally produced, listeners usually notice that the clarity and precision of each frequency (pitch) in the music seem much improved. Engineers who are refining digital technology in hearing aids strive to improve the quality of sound for their listeners as well. Their goal: reduced background noise, improved clarity of speech, and better volume control.

A true all-digital hearing aid is not yet available commercially, but digital technology does exist to suppress background noise in hearing aids. Because a conventional hearing aid can also have a noise-suppression option built in, there may seem to be no difference between conventional and digitally controlled devices. But there is. The distinction lies in the superior way the digital circuitry recognizes noise and manages to separate it from speech. A computer chip capable of making automatic adjustments for loudness and reduction of background noise can be programmed and installed at the factory when a hearing aid is ordered.

Many digitally controlled aids are called *hybrid* hearing aids because they combine conventional (analog) components with certain digital controls. These hybrid devices resemble conventional hearing aids, but they contain a preprogrammed, digitally controlled noise-reduction filter. The way this digitally controlled filter works cannot be changed—or reprogrammed—by its operator or the hearing aid dispenser. If any alteration in the digitally controlled portion of the hearing aid is necessary, the device must be sent back to the factory.

Advantages. These units have circuitry that can be programmed to adapt to the way the unit works in a noisy setting, making it easier for the wearer to understand speech. Also, there may be some improvement in the quality of sound.

Disadvantages. The actual effectiveness of these units, as compared to conventional hearing aids, has received mixed reviews. Some users have reported a small improvement in understanding speech, as long as the talker is speaking in the higher frequencies and the background noise is in the lower frequencies.

If the background noise comes from speech, such as when many people are talking all at once, or if the noise contains a mixture of frequencies, the improvement may be only slight.

Programmable Hearing Aids

A programmable hearing aid, which also employs digital technology, can be programmed by an audiologist or dealer right in the office.

Some of these hearing aids may contain several programs to help the user cope with various hearing problems. The programs are stored in the memory of a microchip located inside the hearing aid. As the wearer's needs change, the dispensing audiologist or dealer can reprogram the hearing aid by using a special piece of computerized office equipment that adjusts the settings.

The various programmable hearing aids that are now available express different theories of sound. For example, one manufacturer offers a programmable hearing aid based on the premise that each person's individual environment contains many different sounds and that he or she responds differently to the acoustics of each listening situation. Accordingly, that hearing aid is designed to amplify particular sound environments in a different way.

Another programmable hearing aid relies on the theory that people respond differently to loudness. This device allows the wearer to hear soft sounds in the environment without being overwhelmed by loud sounds or competing noise.

Another programmable hearing aid is based on the theory of programming the circuitry by individual frequencies. As the user moves from one setting to another, such as from a quiet room into a noisy social gathering, the hearing aid attempts to automatically alter the shape of the amplification for that environment.

Advantages. Programmable hearing aids give you greater flexibility in amplifying the signals. For example, the unit can be reprogrammed based on your personal listening experience. This ability to fine-tune incoming sounds for your individual hearing needs is similar to searching for a station on a stereo receiver: Punching in the number of a station allows you greater precision in locating that station, as opposed to turning the dial randomly until you hit the station.

With this kind of hearing aid, you can work closely with the dispenser to make sure the programming meets your needs. If your hearing changes after you buy the unit, your dispenser can reprogram the device right in his or her office.

Disadvantages. Many of these hearing aids rely on remote-control devices to adjust the hearing aid and change the program. In some cases, the remote control is necessary to turn the unit on and off as well. If you forget or misplace the remote, you can't operate the hearing aid. And if the remote breaks down, you can't use the unit until the remote is repaired or you get a loan of another one.

Another disadvantage is cost. These devices are two to three times higher than conventional hearing aids.

Although these aids feature advanced circuitry and programming intended to reduce noise, their ability to control unwanted sound is far from perfect. Different programs can help to manage sound levels in an especially quiet or noisy area, but gradations vary so much from place to place that the goal of this circuitry has not yet been fully realized. Manufacturers are trying to develop more powerful units, but until they do, many of these hearing aids will not work for people with a more severe degree of hearing loss.

Users may also have to change batteries fairly frequently because digital components use more power. This may cause inconvenience for some.

Many of these units have a *telecoil* or T-coil feature, which allows a hearing aid wearer to use a telephone. However, a few aids may have only a moderately powerful T-switch, which activates the T-coil. Nor do all units have direct audio input, which allows them to be connected to a television, radio, or stereo system.

STYLES OF HEARING AIDS

Vanity has always been a major reason why many hard-of-hearing people don't want to wear a hearing aid. But just as hearing aids have gotten better in terms of technology, they also have become smaller in size—making them more cosmetically acceptable.

In-the-ear, in-the-canal, or behind-the-ear hearing aids are the styles generally available today. Eyeglasses that feature a hearing aid in the glass frames were common decades ago and may be still available, but they are rarely seen today. Body-worn hearing aids are used only for young children and severely hearing-impaired individuals. Depending on the degree and configuration of your hearing loss, you may be able to wear one or more styles of hearing aids. Remember, too, that although some ads may imply that "one size fits all," no one style of hearing aid is appropriate for every type of hearing loss or each individual's special needs.

Some of the bulkier units offer a great deal of flexibility for adding specialized components. For example, a hearing aid that is worn behind the ear can accommodate any or all of the special hearing aid features that are now available. The in-the-ear and in-the canal hearing aids, because of their extremely compact size, may be able to contain only a limited number of special options.

Behind-the-Ear Hearing Aids

Over the past few decades, up until the early eighties, behind-the-ear (BTE) hearing aids were the most popular type of hearing aid sold in the United States. The BTE model, with its arc-like shape (often compared to a large-size shrimp), contains an amplification device that fits neatly behind the ear. (A BTE hearing aid usually doesn't interfere with wearing eyeglasses, either.)

This device conveys sound into the ear canal through a small piece of flexible plastic tubing that connects with a small piece, also plastic, called an earmold. Because of its larger size, a BTE hearing aid can accommodate any or all of the special features that can be built into its circuitry. Its size also enables it to offer more effective amplification and control of incoming sound.

Most children who need a hearing aid are fitted with a BTE model, for several reasons. Its durability makes it an excellent choice for an active child, and these units also offer plenty of flexibility for a growing youngster whose hearing loss changes. Many adults, too, still prefer BTE hearing aids because of their versatility and their overall effectiveness.

This style of listening device also may be somewhat less expensive than other units. Again, cost depends on how much extra circuitry is added to the basic model. The cost of a basic behind-the-ear hearing aid starts at about $500, and can go as high as $2,000 for a programmable model with multiple memory.

Advantages. BTE hearing aids are versatile, durable, and reliable. Their larger size allows for use of a bigger, longer-lasting battery, which is easier to install than a miniature battery. The controls for volume and tone also are easy to manipulate, a feature that is especially helpful for people with limited dexterity in their fingers.

A BTE hearing aid can be used for any degree of hearing loss—from mild to extreme. This kind of unit can be powerful without creating acoustic feedback—the high-pitched squealing or whistling sound that is so annoying to hearing aid wearers.

The earmold portion is easy to keep clean. If you need a new earmold, the only part that needs to be replaced is this one piece of plastic—not the entire hearing aid. Since the electronic components fit behind the ear, not in it, the inner workings are protected from earwax.

Many assistive listening devices are designed to be used with BTE hearing aids (see chapter 6). And it may be easier to obtain a loaner BTE hearing aid from your dispenser if your unit needs to be sent back to the factory for repairs.

Disadvantages. A behind-the-ear hearing aid is more conspicuous, so some hearing-impaired people reject it for cosmetic reasons. Others may consider these devices old-fashioned and not a state-of-the-art product.

People who wear eyeglasses with an oversized temple piece may have difficulty with a BTE hearing aid because it adds to the weight on the top of the outer ear. Also, some people may have ears that are exceptionally close to the head, and a BTE device will not rest easily behind the ear.

The position of the microphone outside the ear minimizes the squeal of acoustic feedback. If you are outdoors in windy weather, however, the microphone may pick up and amplify the whistling of the wind and similar environmental sounds.

In-the-Ear Hearing Aids

The most commonly worn style of hearing aid today is the in-the-ear (ITE) hearing device. The ITE models are fitted with a microphone, amplifier, and speaker. All these components are contained in a small crescent-shaped case that is custom-made to match the contours of your ear just outside the opening of the ear canal.

The ability of manufacturers to miniaturize components and to further improve the durability of ITE hearing aids has added to their appeal. Also, many of these units are now available with programmable controls.

Not too long ago, ITE hearing aids were recommended mainly for people with mild-to-moderate hearing loss. Today, they may be indicated for some people with moderate-to-severe hearing impairment and may be appropriate for some kinds of high-frequency hearing loss as well. Depending on the degree and configuration of your hearing loss, your dispenser may or may not recommend this style of hearing aid for you.

Some ITE hearing aids have a so-called low-profile appearance. This means that the case containing the components is the same size as that of the regular ITE hearing aid, but it has a faceplate that allows the microphone, battery cover, and volume control to be recessed. Thus, the unit is far less visible to the naked eye.

Despite the small size of the ITE units, they can accommodate a surprising number of special features. The price of a standard in-the-ear hearing aid ranges from $550 to $800. Digitally controlled and programmable models are priced significantly higher.

Advantages. ITE units are relatively small in size, but are still visible to others. Because the microphone is located closer to the ear canal, it is thought to deliver sound to the ear in a more natural way. The controls are also fairly easy to adjust.

Disadvantages. This unit may feel uncomfortable in your ear in hot weather. And if you don't have enough dexterity in your fingers or range of motion in your shoulders, it may be difficult to insert the device in your ear properly and adjust the volume control as necessary.

The smaller size limits the amount of amplification and power the unit is capable of producing. Acoustic feedback, or constant squealing, can be a problem because the microphone and the receiver are fitted very close together within the plastic case.

The ear canal may feel a bit plugged when using this style. If you have an especially small ear canal and canal opening, you may not be able to wear an ITE hearing aid.

In-the-Canal Hearing Aids

Most adults today who go to buy a hearing aid want an in-the-canal (ITC) model, also known as a canal aid. Advertising has had a clear impact on the demand for these markedly less visible devices, but manufacturers' claims that canal-type hearing aids are "invisible" just aren't true.

ITC hearing aids fit entirely into the space at the beginning of the ear canal. Cosmetically, these hearing aids are small and discreet. Acoustically, they're limited by the amount of power, flexibility, and range of frequencies they can pick up.

If you have mild-to-moderate hearing loss, you may be a good candidate for an ITC hearing aid. Some sales pitches tout the ability of canal hearing aids to improve all levels of hearing loss, but at this point these units still lack the power to provide good amplification without acoustic feedback.

The price of an ITC hearing aid ranges from $1,200 to $2,000.

Advantages. This unit is the least visible of all the hearing aid styles.

Disadvantages. Despite increased efforts at further miniaturization of the electronic components, limited volume remains a major drawback of these units. To compound this problem, when additional power is built into an ITC hearing aid, it increases the chance of acoustic feedback. Unwanted noise also may be hard to keep out, because these tiny hearing aids remain too small to incorporate a sufficient number of filters to suppress noise.

After wearing an ITC device all day, some people may find that over a period of time the hearing aid begins to feel uncomfortable.

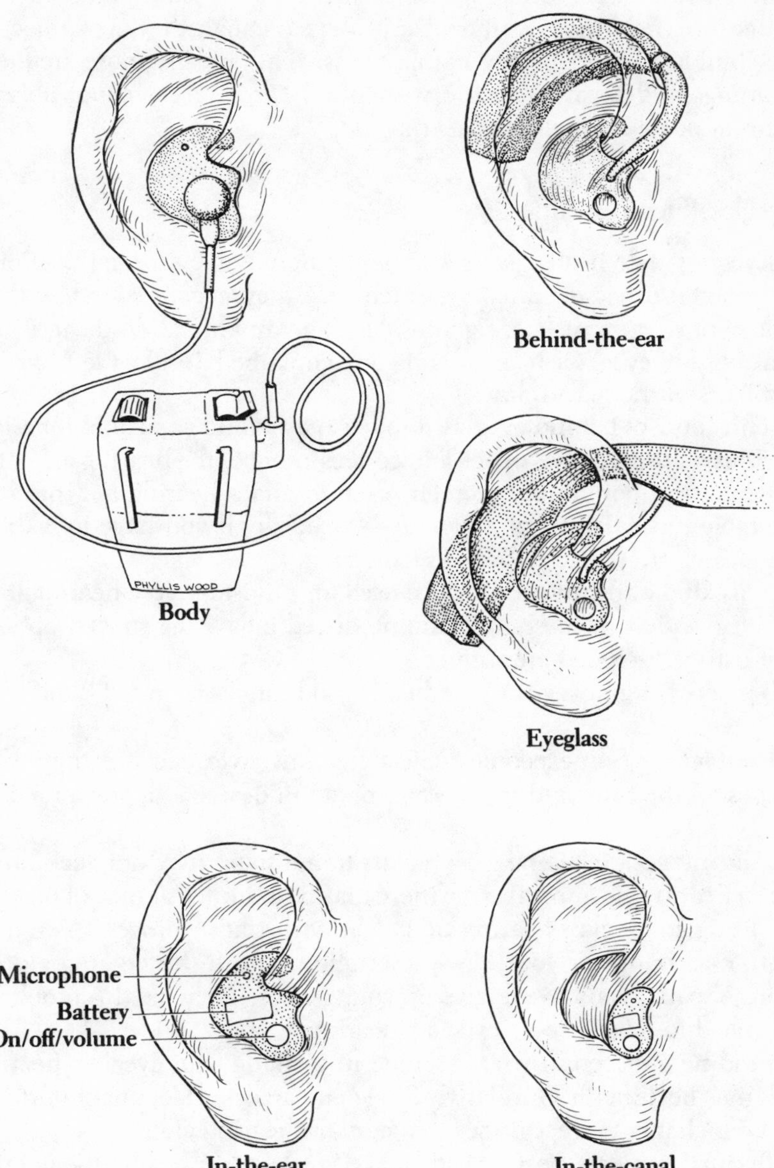

Examples of hearing-aid styles

The small size of the units makes them difficult to handle for people with arthritic finger joints, limited dexterity, and vision problems.

Because these models sit deeper in the ear canal, they are subject to wax buildup on their tiny components. This means more frequent cleanings and repairs. People with small ear canals are not able to accommodate a canal-style hearing aid.

Eyeglass Hearing Aids

Eyeglass-style hearing aids were a popular choice during the 1960s, but their use has declined so much that they account for less than 1 percent of current hearing aid sales. The amplification devices and controls for eyeglass hearing aids are contained inside the bows or earpieces of the glass frames.

The concept behind eyeglass models may sound appealing for a few obvious reasons: convenience and concealment of the hearing aid components. But combining corrective lenses and a hearing aid into one wearable piece can be problematic—especially if you have to take off the glasses or chance to break a lens.

This kind of hearing aid can be used for mild-to-severe hearing loss. Because so few of these units are produced today, the special options that can be included are limited.

The cost of an eyeglass-style hearing aid ranges from $700 to $850.

Advantages. Some people may prefer this style because they wear glasses all the time and see the combination device as a convenience.

Disadvantages. The newer eyeglass frame styles may not accommodate a hearing aid apparatus, so there may be a limited choice of frames.

Fitting an eyeglass hearing aid can be a frustrating process. You may require a change of your lens prescription, and if the hearing aid requires repairs, you have to give up your glasses. To avoid this problem, you need to have a spare eyeglass hearing aid on hand.

Finding a dispenser who is skilled in working with eyeglass hearing aids may be difficult. Similarly, some opticians may feel uncomfortable making changes in eyeglasses that contain hearing aids.

Because eyeglass hearing aids make your glasses heavy, they create added pressure on the bridge of your nose. Also, the fit of the eyeglasses against the side of your head may be less snug than you prefer because the bows aren't as flexible as those in regular glasses.

What Will Your Money Buy?

Price	*What You Can Get*
$500–$700	A fairly good behind-the-ear conventional aid, with a 30-day follow-up visit, a six-month checkup, and a one-year warranty. At the high end of this range, you may be able to purchase an in-the-ear aid. If your hearing loss falls in the mild-to-moderate range and your listening environment doesn't vary a lot, this is a good choice.
$700–$1,000	A behind-the-ear aid with several options or an in-the-ear or in-the-canal aid. (The smallest and most expensive are called mini-canal aids.) You'll find that most aids with automatic signal processing (such as the K-Amp circuitry) are in this range. Don't add options you don't need. For example, many people with mild hearing loss won't benefit much from T-coil circuitry.
$1,000–$1,200	A conventional aid with several options or one of the lower cost digital aids. You should consider a digital aid if your hearing loss is moderate to severe, if you change listening environments frequently, or if conventional aids have not worked well for you.
$1,200–$2,000	A behind-the-ear or in-the-ear digitally programmed aid.

The prices given are typical ranges, determined by information from manufacturers and several audiologists. Prices, which vary by region, are generally higher in large urban areas than in small towns. But since prices vary fairly widely even within the same region, it pays to shop around. The dispenser should offer a better deal if you are buying an aid for each ear (a binaural fitting).

CROS Hearing Aids

A CROS (contralateral routing of signals) hearing aid is recommended when you have a significant hearing loss in one ear but good hearing in the other ear.

When both ears have a hearing loss, and an audiologist has determined that you would benefit by using two hearing aids, you would most probably have a *binaural fitting*. But some people with significant asymmetry in their hearing loss find no real benefit to wearing a hearing aid in their worse ear. CROS hearing aids have two earpieces that work together as a single unit. A microphone is placed in the weaker ear to pick up sound and transmit it to the stronger ear, allowing that ear to do most of the hearing.

In the past, a wire worn behind the head or built into eyeglass hearing aids was used to transmit sound from one side of the head to the other. Wireless transmission is possible today by means of FM radio frequencies that have been reserved for this purpose.

A CROS hearing aid may be recommended for some people who have had a sudden loss of hearing from an infection or accident, mainly because they were accustomed to stereo reception of sound before losing their hearing. A CROS hearing aid doesn't produce stereo input, but it does allow you to pick up sounds around both sides of your head.

A BICROS hearing aid is a variation on the CROS. This type of aid is used when the better ear has some degree of hearing impairment and also requires amplification.

HEARING AID OPTIONS

Numerous options, or special features, are available for certain styles of hearing aids. Although some are standard items, most of these special-order add-ons can substantially increase the cost of a hearing aid.

These extras offer better control of the sounds you hear through the hearing aid and include custom built-ins such as filters, switches, or special circuits. Not every type of hearing loss requires each of these features, and not every style of hearing aid can accommodate each of these options. The larger the hearing aid, the more features that can be packed into the unit. Some of these extras are beneficial to some wearers, but take care not to add options that you don't need.

Among these available options are:

- *Tone control.* This control modifies the sensitivity of the amplifier inside the hearing aid. Depending on the type of device, you may be able to adjust for low-frequency sounds, high-frequency sounds, or both. The tone control allows you to amplify higher frequencies, such as speech, and minimize lower frequencies that may interfere with your understanding of speech. Your audiologist or dealer can adjust the hearing aid to emphasize the frequency range that is most useful for you.
- *Feedback control.* This control reduces the squeal or whistling noise of acoustic feedback that is produced when the hearing aid's microphone and receiver are very close to each other. Hearing aids with stronger amplification and those that are designed to emphasize the higher frequencies tend to be more prone to feedback.
- *Output or power control.* A power control differs from volume control, which comes as standard equipment on every hearing aid. By setting the power control a certain way, your dispenser can vary the power and amplification your hearing aid produces. This allows you to run the unit at full strength when necessary, or to lower it and thus conserve your batteries.

  If you have bought a stronger hearing aid than you need, or your hearing changes and you require more power, this control allows you to increase the power without having to buy a new aid.
- *Compression circuits.* If you are highly sensitive to loud sounds, it is important that your hearing aid doesn't amplify noise above a tolerable level. A compression circuit will decrease the volume (gain) that a hearing aid produces when the volume level of the environment increases around you.

  This control works to protect your ears by automatically compressing sound to a lower level as soon as the volume reaches a certain intensity. When the noise in the environment decreases, the compression circuit shuts itself off.

  There are a few different kinds of compression circuits: automatic gain control, input and output compression, and frequency-dependent compression. The proper choice depends on your individual needs.
- *Adaptive circuits to reduce noise.* These circuits are called automatic signal processing or noise suppression controls, and are

Extras for Your Hearing Aid

Option	Cost*	Description
Push-Pull Circuit/Power Circuit/Power Pak/Linear Plus	$50	Powerful hearing aid circuitry used to correct very severe hearing loss
Automatic Signal Processing	$50–$80	Circuitry that helps reduce distortion caused by background noise, by amplifying low-frequency sounds less than the higher-frequency sounds of conversation
Telecoil	$50	Circuitry that picks up electromagnetic radiation from telephones; helps people talk on the telephone without feedback; used mainly in behind-the-ear aids
Compression	$40–$50	Feature that keeps loud sounds from being overamplified
Automatic Gain Control (AGC)	$100–$150	Circuitry that helps control distortion and interference caused by background noise and keeps loud sounds from becoming uncomfortably loud; allows the wearer to move between different listening situations—from a car to a noisy party, for example—without adjusting the volume of the aid

K-Amp	\$100–\$200	Circuitry that amplifies soft-to-medium sounds without amplifying loud sounds
Output Control/MPO	\$200	Amplifies circuitry that allows the dispenser to adjust how loud sounds can get
Remote Control	\$400–\$900	Device for digital aids that allows you to switch between preprogrammed settings for different listening situations; one setting for watching television, for example, and another for attending a football game; often included as a part of the package price

*Figures represent cost to dispenser; cost to consumer may be somewhat higher. Costs are averages and vary from brand to brand.

intended to reduce distortion and interference produced by background noise. They also make it easier to understand speech.

A newer variation on this is the patented *K-Amp* circuitry that amplifies soft speech sounds without also making louder background sounds more intense. Hearing aids that contain the K-Amp cannot be customized as precisely as digitally programmed models. Instead, this option is geared to the most common problem associated with hearing loss: It selectively boosts the amplification of quiet sounds and high-frequency sounds. People with mild hearing loss often do well with a K-Amp, although those with moderate-to-severe hearing loss may find that this feature doesn't amplify the low frequencies enough for them to hear clearly. Though K-Amp hearing aids are less costly than digital ones, they don't come cheap. According to the company that licenses the

K-Amp, hearing aids containing this amplifier cost $700 to $900—$100 to $200 more than their traditional counterparts.

- *Push-pull circuitry and dual receivers*. This kind of circuitry is intended for an individual with severe hearing loss. These options allow increased power and amplification without distorting the quality and clarity of the sound. By having two receivers instead of one, circuit overload is prevented.
- *Telecoil (T-coil)*. Telecoil circuitry allows you to hear conversations on the telephone more effectively while using a hearing aid. You flip a T-switch to activate this circuitry as you need it. When the switch is on, the hearing aid stops amplifying sound waves and instead amplifies the electromagnetic waves produced in the telephone receiver. This feature eliminates the acoustic feedback many people experience when they use conventional hearing aids with a telephone, and it helps shut out background noise.

  Behind-the-ear and eyeglass-style hearing aids usually offer a T-coil as a standard item. It is available as an option for in-the-ear hearing aids, but a canal-style hearing aid cannot accommodate this feature.

  Before ordering a T-coil, do a little research. The quality and strength of telecoil circuitry varies from manufacturer to manufacturer. Also, certain T-coils work better with some telephones than others. If you are considering a T-coil, ask your dispenser if you can try out different ones before you order your hearing aid. And be sure to check with the local office of your telephone company to make sure that the phone you use is compatible with T-coil circuitry.

  The law now requires all public telephones and new models of home telephones to be compatible with telecoil circuitry. If you are buying a new phone, check the label on the box. Some retailers may still be carrying old stock.

  A telephone switch on a hearing aid also allows the wearer to hook up with other assistive listening devices, including the loop system used in many auditoriums, houses of worship, and concert halls.
- *Direct audio input*. Direct audio input allows a hearing aid to connect directly with a television, stereo system, or radio for amplification of the sound, while at the same time decreasing background noise. This feature is mainly available in behind-the-ear styles.

- *Digitally controlled and programmable circuitry.* Digital circuitry uses the same technology that is available to program the microchips of computers. This technology converts the electrical signals entering a hearing aid's microphone into numbers, then modifies them as directed by a computer program stored inside the hearing aid. Once modified, the signals are converted back into sound that is transferred into the receiver for entry into the ear. This option, such as the Automatic Gain Control (AGC), may offer better noise control and more exact correction of your hearing loss.

  With further refinements in the applications of digital technology, it is expected that digital circuitry will eventually come into common use among hearing aid wearers.

HOW TO CHOOSE A HEARING AID

Before even considering the purchase of a hearing aid, you should first have your hearing evaluated by a physician. This will rule out any underlying disease or medical problem that may be causing hearing loss.

If you do not have a problem that can be treated medically or surgically, the hearing specialist will recommend a hearing aid evaluation by an audiologist. By using a battery of tests, including speech reception threshold and speech discrimination (see chapter 3), the audiologist assesses your ability to hear and to understand speech both with and without a hearing aid. Another aspect of testing and diagnosis that is critical for hearing aid candidates is tolerance testing.

Tolerance Testing

If it has been determined that you would benefit from using a hearing aid, this important test *must* be performed during the hearing aid evaluation. Tolerance testing determines the level at which you find it comfortable to listen to speech, as well as the level at which speech becomes so uncomfortably loud that you find it intolerable.

By ascertaining your level of discomfort, the audiologist can preset your hearing aid so that it never reaches that level. You also may be asked to sample and compare a variety of hearing aids. Based upon the results of the tolerance test and your comments about the various hearing devices, the audiologist will recommend a hearing aid that will best serve your individual needs.

Before You Buy . . .
Some Consumer Guidelines

Many consumers who buy hearing aids derive no benefit from their purchase because they never really needed a hearing aid in the first place. Typically, they went to a dealer and chose a hearing aid without first seeking a medical evaluation. Many may have found, too late, that they have a problem that could have been corrected by medical or surgical treatment. Or perhaps they took a salesperson's advice and made a purchase that they soon regretted.

Bad experiences with hearing aids and the people who sell them are common. That's why it's important to be wary of advertisements that downplay the need for a medical examination and a hearing evaluation.

Aware of the many scams and frauds connected with hearing aid sales, the FDA requires that a licensed physician evaluate your hearing within six months prior to purchase of a hearing aid, unless you sign a waiver. Some dispensers may encourage you to sign this waiver, which states that you agree to give up your right to a medical examination. FDA regulations also require dispensers and dealers to advise you that forgoing a medical examination is not in your best interests.

The sale of hearing aids to those under age 18 is subject to federal safeguards. If a child needs a hearing aid, a medical examination and audiological test must always be performed before a dispenser can fit that child with a hearing device.

Because adults have no such legal protection, the old rule of thumb applies especially to hearing aid purchases: Let the buyer beware.

Which Hearing Aid Is Right for You?

From an audiologist's perspective, the most important considerations in recommending a hearing aid include efficiency, durability, service record, purchase price, operating price, and appearance—in that order.

But if you are like most people faced with the selection of a hearing aid, cosmetic considerations such as size and appearance of the device most likely will be your primary concern. Cost also may be a major issue.

In selecting the right hearing aid, the dispenser's goal is to choose an instrument that will provide you with the best understanding of speech in the greatest number of possible situations. To achieve that goal, you may be urged to choose a certain kind of hearing aid, such as a behind-the-ear model. If you reject this recommendation and insist on a smaller, more cosmetically acceptable device, you can expect to compromise the benefits you will get from the aid.

Your hearing aid evaluation may show that you would benefit by wearing not just one but two hearing aids, or a binaural fitting. Wearing two hearing aids can enhance the ability to sense where sound is coming from and to hear equally from both sides. The downside is cost. If you are considering a binaural fitting, it is perfectly acceptable to ask your dispenser for a discount on the second device. In most cases, the dealer will make an allowance for the second hearing aid. If not, you may want to find a recommended dispenser who will give you a price break for buying two units.

Now that many states require a 30-day trial period for hearing aids, some dispensers advise new users to order two hearing aids and then to decide whether they want to keep both or just one.

FINDING A RELIABLE DEALER

Historically, sellers of hearing aids have earned their place among the variety of snake-oil salesmen who peddle their products by using pressure tactics to sell questionable merchandise.

Even today, despite federal and state regulations designed to protect hearing aid buyers (and the development of industry standards for providers), consumers still need to be cautious in choosing a dispenser.

Trust and reliability are critical issues in making the right choice of a provider of hearing devices. When you purchase a hearing aid, you are not just buying an appliance and taking it home. You are also choosing someone who will teach you how to use your hearing aid, provide regular servicing for the unit, and work with you on a continuing basis to help you get the best use of your aid.

Several resources exist in most communities for checking out hearing aid dispensers, such as the Better Business Bureau, local consumer protection groups, and your state attorney general's office. In addition, you may want to check with the licensing board for hearing aid dispensers located in your state capital. Inquire as to whether there are any complaints on file about any of the dispensers you are considering and, if so, how they were resolved. Check credentials carefully: Some dealers have been known to pass themselves off as audiologists or even as medical doctors.

In order to be licensed in most states, a dispenser of hearing aids must meet certain standards of competence and follow a strict code of ethics. The International Hearing Society (IHS), a nonprofit trade group previously known as the National Hearing Aid Society, has a voluntary certification program for its members. To earn board certification from this professional trade organization, a dispenser must take a certain amount of continuing education courses. When a dealer is certified by the National Board of Certification of Hearing Instrument Sciences, the letters *BC-HIS* are displayed by the dealer's name.

Dispensing audiologists are audiologists who are specially trained to fit people with hearing aids. Many states require that audiologists be licensed. The professional association that certifies these providers and regulates their educational requirements is the American Speech-Language-Hearing Association (ASHA). ASHA requires that any of its members who provide clinical services also apply for and obtain a certificate of clinical competence in audiology. When the letters CCC-A follow an audiologist's name, it indicates that this nonphysician specialist has obtained certification.

Both of these groups—IHS and ASHA—can provide the names of qualified hearing aid fitters and dispensers in your area. (See appendix B for addresses and telephone numbers.)

Some localities, particularly rural ones, may have no audiologists nearby, and you may have to go directly to a recommended hearing aid dealer. Dealers have less formal education than audiologists, and generally use more limited diagnostic equipment than audiologists do. Still, they may have a great deal of practical experience in fitting hearing aids, and can be quite competent.

After obtaining the names of dispensers, call and arrange a visit. Meet them, get price quotes, and learn their customer service policies. Doing this kind of groundwork allows you to develop a sense of what it would be like to work with this person in the months and years to come. You need to know that you are getting the best price for the hearing aid you plan to buy, but more important, you must feel that you can trust the dispenser and value the advice and counsel you will receive.

Questions to Ask

Consider your first meeting with the dispenser as an interview in which you have the opportunity to get all the information you need. Among the questions you should be prepared to ask are:

- How long have you been in business?
- Are you a certified member of the International Hearing Society or the American Speech-Language-Hearing Association?
- Do you sell only one brand or several? (Avoid dispensers who sell only one brand or type of hearing aid. No manufacturer makes a hearing aid that's right for everyone. To achieve the optimum fit, your dispenser should have a wide variety of aids to choose from.)
- Which models and brands of hearing aid can best meet my listening needs? Why are you recommending a particular brand or brands? How long have these particular manufacturers been in business? Are hearing aids and electronics their main business? (If your audiologist has recommended a particular brand or brands, look for a dealer who sells and services this particular brand.)
- Do you service the hearing aids that you sell? Is there a qualified repairperson on the premises, or must the hearing aid be sent elsewhere for repair work?
- Do you offer a 30-day trial period during which time I can return the hearing aid if I'm not satisfied? (In some states, a trial period is mandated by law; check your local regulations.) Is the trial period free, or am I required to pay an extra fee for this protection? If so, what is the fee?
- What is the total cost of the hearing aid I'm considering? Will you provide me with a written quote? Exactly what is included in this price?
- If I buy two hearing aids, what will it cost? Are you willing to give me a discount for the second hearing aid?
- What services are included in the price of the hearing aid? (Some dispensers provide special training, known as aural rehabilitation, to help you adjust to your hearing aid and make the best use of it.

This valuable training shows you how to use visual cues such as facial expressions and lip movements.)

- If I have a problem with my hearing aid, can I just drop by your office or do I need to call to schedule an appointment?
- If my hearing changes, what kind of testing and related equipment do you have on the premises? Is the person who runs this equipment a trained technician, a dispenser with some training, or a dispensing audiologist?
- Make sure the dispenser has the means to perform a real ear measurement test, which experts say is essential to getting a well-fitted and operating hearing aid (see page 112).

It's helpful to take written notes during each visit to a dispenser. Invite a family member or friend to accompany you. Besides offering support, this person may be able to take notes while you ask questions or inquire about something you may have overlooked.

Regardless of how persuasive, persistent, or pressuring a dispenser may be, don't sign a contract, make a down payment, or feel compelled to buy a hearing aid on the spot. If the dispenser tries to tempt you by mentioning a "special sale," ask how long this sale is running. If the response is that "it ends today," that may be true—or it may be a gimmick to push you to buy.

Once you have obtained the facts you need from the first dispenser you are considering, visit the next one, ask the same questions, and get a price quote. After comparison shopping, you can intelligently assess this information and then decide where you want to buy your hearing aid.

Again, purchasing a hearing aid is a package deal in which you are paying for the product you choose as well as for the dispenser's expertise and services. Experience, reputation, skill, training, and available services are key areas to consider in making your choice. Another consideration is cost. As you comparison-shop, you may find that the quoted price for a hearing aid may differ by several hundred dollars, depending on the dealer. Try to balance this difference with the services provided and the reputation of the dealer when making your choice.

The Trial Period

Most hearing aid dispensers provide a trial period during which time you can return the instrument if you are not satisfied. The laws in many states require that consumers receive at least a 30-day trial period.

This trial may be free or carry a small service fee that can vary from 5 to 20 percent of the purchase price.

Whatever the fee, get this figure in writing as a part of your price quote. Dispensers should be willing to apply this fee to the purchase price if you decide to keep the hearing aid. If the instrument proves to

Door-to-Door and Mail-Order Sales of Hearing Aids

Just as it is not advisable to buy a hearing aid from a suitcase in a salesperson's car trunk, it is also risky to do so through the mail. These hearing aids are usually overpriced and may be lacking in quality. The FTC has identified some of the deceptive advertisements that often appear about hearing aids. The most common include:

- Direct or implied representations that hearing aids will help every person in every situation.
- An advertisement in the print or broadcast media stating that you'll receive a "free gift" or "free valuable information" without also mentioning that a salesperson will visit you at home.
- Promising you a "free replica of a hearing aid," which is actually a nonworking piece of plastic that a salesperson delivers to your home.

If you happen to buy a hearing aid from an itinerant salesperson, you have the right under the FTC's Door-to-Door Sales Rule to cancel within three days for any sale of $25 or more. This rule applies to sales that occur in your home or at a location that is not the seller's regular place of business.

Federal law does not ban the mail-order sale of hearing aids, but several states have outlawed this kind of transaction. In the states that permit hearing aid sales by mail, each order is subject to the FTC's Mail Order Rule. This requires that a company ship each purchase when promised—or give consumers the option to cancel their order for a refund.

be unsatisfactory and you return it, you may have to forfeit some or all of the service fee you paid in advance.

Most dispensers will want to see you at least twice during the 30-day trial period. The purpose of the trial is to give you the opportunity to wear the hearing aid, experiment with it, have it readjusted if you're not pleased with it, or return it and select a different unit. If the hearing aid doesn't meet your needs, you can either ask the dealer to remedy the problem, or you can request a refund. Whatever you do, be sure to act within the 30-day period.

Keep copies of all your documents, including your purchase agreement and receipts, in case there is a problem. If a dispenser fails to make any mention of a trial period, and balks when you ask about it, find another dispenser.

The Purchase Agreement

After comparing prices and dispensers and deciding who you want to deal with, it's important to carefully review your contract, or purchase agreement, which spells out the terms of the transaction. This document should clearly explain in writing each verbal promise that was made to you. The terms of the 30-day trial period should also be noted on this agreement.

Terms of payment need to be explained carefully before you sign a purchase agreement. A dispenser may ask for a down payment upon placing your order and require payment in full when you receive the hearing aid. Others may ask for the balance at the conclusion of your trial period. If you aren't comfortable with a dispenser's payment policy, see what other dispensers have to offer.

If you decide to cancel your purchase during the trial period, your dispenser may retain a portion of your deposit as a nonrefundable fitting charge to cover the cost of ordering your custom-fit earmold. Dispensers who administer hearing evaluation tests and defer the billing until giving you an invoice for your hearing aid can also charge you for the cost of these tests if you cancel.

Read the fine print of your purchase agreement to see if the dealer has a "restocking fee" or a "dispensing fee," which is analogous to the dealer surcharge added to some new cars. If so, be aware that cancellation means that you must pay this excessive, nonrefundable fee.

Be certain that you understand all of the details of your contract before you sign or make a down payment. Among the points to consider in reviewing your contract are:

- Will I receive a written warranty? Who honors the warranty—the dispenser, the manufacturer, or both? Are you a factory-authorized dealer for the brand of hearing aid I am purchasing? (Some manufacturers may not recognize warranties unless their product was purchased from an authorized seller of their brand.)
- What services will you provide free of charge, and how long will this arrangement last?
- If my hearing aid requires repairs, will you provide a loaner unit?
- Is the 30-day trial period free? If there is a charge, exactly how much must I pay for this service? Will this fee be applied to the purchase price if I buy the hearing aid? Will you please clearly note that in writing on the contract?
- What is your policy on returns and exchanges?
- If I choose to sign an installment credit contract to pay for the hearing aid, what are the finance charges? How is this reflected as an annual percentage rate, and what is the total cost of carrying this credit?

Hearing aid professionals and providers have found that good performance by a hearing aid in a clinical setting doesn't necessarily mean the device will serve you as well elsewhere. To complicate matters, often there is only a slight difference in performance among hearing aids—a problem that makes selection of a particular model especially difficult.

The Department of Veterans Affairs (VA) tests and evaluates dozens of hearing aid models each year, alternating custom-made, in-the-ear models one year, and regular "stock" models (including on-the-body, over-the-ear, and eyeglass units) the next. While their top-rated models aren't necessarily best for each individual, the test results may be useful to your audiologist (see appendix A).

You can obtain a summary of the results by writing to Audiology and Speech/Language Pathology Service, Department of Veterans Affairs Medical Center, 50 Irving Street N.W., Washington, DC 20422.

For further information about hearing loss and hearing aids, call the Better Hearing Institute's toll-free line (1-800-EARWELL). Or write the Consumer Affairs Department of the American Association of Retired Persons (AARP), 1909 K Street N.W., Washington, DC 20049.

FITTING AND OPERATING A HEARING AID

Glasses are prescribed based on the scientific measurement and diagnosis of the ability of each of your eyes to focus on an object. The criteria for fitting you with a hearing aid aren't as precise. A dispenser who fine-tunes your hearing aid to best meet your needs must work both with the objective test data from your hearing evaluation and any subjective information that you offer about your hearing experiences.

In fact, the word *fitting* has a few different applications when used to discuss hearing aids. In one sense, fitting a hearing aid means that your dispenser is adjusting the instrument to your specific hearing needs. This includes advising you which model and special circuitry are best for you. If an audiologist thinks that a behind-the-ear hearing aid would give you optimum results, but you want a smaller canal-style unit, discussing this issue is a part of the fitting procedure.

Fitting also refers to the actual physical fitting of the hearing aid in your ear.

Which Brand Is Best?

There is no simple way to tell in advance which of the many brands of hearing aid will work best for a given person. Individual patterns of hearing loss are different, and the optimal model for one person may be less than ideal for someone else. (That's why hearing aids sold through mail-order catalogs without individual testing—a new marketing trend—are likely to be ineffective or even harmful.) The best strategy is to go to an audiologist or hearing aid dealer who can let you try several different models to find the best fit and the best value.

Two hearing aid manufacturers—*Miracle Ear* and *Beltone*—now advertise their products directly to consumers. *Miracle Ear* spent $5.5 million on cable television advertising last year alone. Despite what their ads may lead you to believe, however, these companies make products similar to those available from a number of manufacturers; it's only the marketing approach that's different. When you call the toll-free number in the ads, the company takes down your name and telephone number and sells it to a local distributor for about $30. The local shop then contacts you for an appointment.

If you go to a one-brand shop, you could easily end up paying more for a hearing aid than you would for an identical device elsewhere. *Miracle Ear*, for example, buys some of its behind-the-ear aids from another big name in the hearing aid business, *Oticon*. But while one aid sells for about $700 under the *Oticon* brand name, *Miracle Ear*'s version costs around $1,400.

Often, hearing aid dealers or audiologists will pool their resources and form a buying group to purchase hearing aids from major manufacturers and sell them under a private label. (*Marcon* is a label used by one of the larger buying groups.) By buying in volume, members of the group get name-brand aids at one-third to one-half the cost. Such private labels can be a money-saving option, but only if you buy from a dealer who passes the savings on to the consumer.

Even a dealer who offers a variety of brands may still be partial to the manufacturer who's offering a trip to Hawaii for selling a certain number of its products. Ultimately, the best protection is to shop around. Ask up front if you can pay for your exam and get a copy of your results before you actually buy a hearing aid. That way you can take your results to another dealer or audiologist for a second opinion on the type of hearing aid that would be best for you.

The Physical Fit

The initial step of the physical fitting centers around creating the earmold, the custom-made plastic piece that enters your outer ear. Earmolds help to anchor the hearing aid, but more important, their design conducts amplified sound waves into the ear and affects the quality of the sound you hear. There are many different types and styles of earmolds. The size of the earmold that is chosen for you is based on your hearing loss. A significant degree of hearing loss usually requires a larger earmold. Behind-the-ear and eyeglass hearing aids use earmolds that are connected to the aid with clear plastic tubing, which must be replaced when it hardens or turns yellow.

To make an earmold, a puttylike material is placed in your ear canal for several minutes and is allowed to harden. During the short time it remains in your ear, it makes an impression of your ear canal and the surrounding area. The impression is then sent to a laboratory that makes earmolds.

Earmolds are made from hard acrylic plastic and soft vinyl rubber. Some people may develop a sensitivity to either of these materials. If you develop an irritation on the skin in your ear, such as red spots, open sores, or soreness, stop wearing the earmold and contact your dispenser at once. If it is determined that you are having an allergic reaction, then a new earmold can be ordered that is made from a different material.

When the fit is good, you should feel that the earmold or hearing aid is anchored securely in your ear—snug, but not uncomfortably tight. It should not dislodge or fall out when you turn your head. Although you can expect to feel the sensation of something in your ear, it should not be painful. If there are any imperfections, such as rough edges, your dealer can grind down and smooth out these areas for you.

It's important to wear the aid for a while in the dispenser's office or store. It may feel comfortable for the first few minutes, but after wearing the earmold or hearing aid for a longer period, you may find that it is tight or presses too hard in certain areas. When adjustments fail to correct the problem, the dispenser should take another impression and give you an earmold that better fits your ear.

When an earmold or hearing aid has the room to move even slightly in your ear canal, it can result in the whistling or squealing sound of acoustic feedback when you turn up the volume. If this is a problem, you may require a new earmold.

During the first days or weeks of wearing a new hearing aid, you may feel that your ear is plugged. Eventually, you'll become less conscious of your hearing aid and even learn to forget that it's in your ear.

Using a Hearing Aid

When your hearing aid arrives and you go to pick it up, your dispenser will spend some time teaching you how to use it. Training in the proper use of a hearing aid is a vital part of the package of services you have purchased from your dispenser. Keep in mind that you are paying for this instruction and that you are entitled to a reasonable amount of the dispenser's time in learning how to operate your hearing aid correctly.

After checking the physical fit of the hearing aid in your ear, the dispenser will show you how to operate the unit and how to use any of the special features you have ordered. Points that the dispenser should cover include:

- *Proper insertion and removal.* The dispenser should tell you, for example, to make sure that the hearing aid is turned off during insertion to prevent unpleasant feedback noise.
- *How to turn your hearing aid on and off.* As you become familiar with this switch, you should be able to maneuver it quickly.
- *Adjustment of the volume controls.* A hearing aid's volume control turns in one direction or another. However, as you learn how to operate it on a daily basis, you may find adjustments in sound are easier to make simply by listening to whether the sound gets louder or softer.
- *How to use the telephone when you are wearing your hearing aid.* There are two ways to do this—by effectively using the microphone in your hearing aid, or by using a telecoil, or T-switch, feature on your hearing aid.
- *Changing the batteries.* The dispenser will show you the location and the proper way of opening and closing the battery door. There should be a demonstration of how to remove the battery as well as how to replace it. Make note of the correct battery size, and keep extra batteries on hand at all times.
- *Cleaning and caring for your hearing aid.* (See page 114 for additional information.)
- *Setting up a schedule for your aural rehabilitation program.* This program will train you to pick out speech against a variety of background noises. It also should teach you how to sharpen your awareness of visual cues to further enhance what you hear.

No two people adjust to a hearing aid at the same pace. Some wearers may adapt automatically to hearing sound in this new way. Others may take a long time to adjust to the device. Getting accustomed to hearing amplified sound through an instrument and working with your dispenser to make the necessary adjustments are integral to the entire process.

Aided Hearing Test

In addition to your subjective responses to the dispenser's questions, he or she must verify that your hearing aid is properly set and that it corrects or improves your type of hearing loss. To objectively obtain this information, the dispenser administers what is called an *aided hearing test*, which is undertaken while you are wearing the device.

Two kinds of testing are performed—functional gain testing and real ear measurement.

Functional gain testing. This is similar to the tone and speech testing that is done during an audiological workup, but instead of wearing earphones, you wear your hearing aid. The way you respond to each sound or word reflects your level of hearing. Using your test results, the dispenser adjusts the controls on your hearing aid until the equipment measures the best correction of your hearing loss.

Real ear measurement. In this test, a miniature microphone is placed in your ear canal to measure sounds. These are introduced through a loudspeaker. The measurement is taken both with and without the hearing aid in place.

This device actually allows the dispenser to learn how the sound is resonating and being amplified within your ear canal. The information it produces gives the dispenser a better understanding of how the signal should be changed to suit your individual hearing needs. Real ear testing may show that the shape of the earmold or the hearing aid itself must be changed to help modify the incoming sound signals.

Hearing aid scientists have designated real ear measurements as essential to confirm that a hearing aid is working the way it should. Nevertheless, many hearing aid dealers lack the equipment necessary to perform this test. When you first interview hearing aid dispensers, inquire if they have the means to perform this important test.

HOW TO USE A HEARING AID: A LIFETIME PURCHASE

How well your hearing improves as you begin to wear a hearing aid depends on a number of variables: the amount and type of your hearing loss, the listening situations that prove challenging or difficult, your attitude about wearing the device, and your expectations.

Unlike other purchases that you bring home and put away until needed, a hearing aid is meant to be worn regularly every day—even when you spend most of your day at home alone. Consistent use during the first weeks after purchase also helps you to learn how to use the instrument more effectively.

You will have to get used to certain aspects of wearing a hearing aid, such as the feel of the device in your ear and the way it amplifies common sounds. If you have been experiencing a slowly progressing hearing loss, you may even have forgotten what some of the surrounding environment sounds like.

Typical comments of first-time hearing aid wearers include "Flushing the toilet is like standing next to Niagara Falls"; "Silverware falling into a stainless steel sink crashes like thunder"; and "Crunching into an apple sounds like cutting through metal."

It's true that some environmental sounds are amplified more than others, and it takes some time to adjust to these sounds. But only by familiarizing yourself with how things sound through your hearing aid can you learn how to better tune them out by properly adjusting the controls.

Some audiologists and dealers advise customers at first to wear the hearing aid for as long as it feels comfortable in the ear. During the first week, you may be able to wear it for only a few hours a day. Try to gradually increase the amount of time you keep the hearing aid in your ear. (*Note:* When the hearing aid is in your ear, be sure to turn it *on*. Otherwise, the device blocks the entry of incoming sound and diminishes your ability to hear even more.)

Again, it's important not to waste your trial period. Wear your hearing aid. Practice using it in all situations. During this time, bring any problems you have to the dispenser's attention. Most dispensers will ask you to come back after you have had the hearing aid for 10 days to two weeks. Some may also call you during this period to see how you're doing.

Your first return visit gives you the opportunity to tell the dispenser whether something is amiss with the hearing aid. You also can ask for additional instruction if you feel uncomfortable with certain aspects of the hearing aid.

Remember, you are entitled to a 30-day trial period—even if there is a problem with the hearing aid, the fitting, or if you change your mind and decide to buy a different model. If the hearing aid or the earmold is found to be faulty and needs to be sent back for replacement, the time it takes to get a new unit from the factory or laboratory should not be considered a part of the trial period. The same rule applies if you decide that a different hearing aid would work better for you, and you want to exchange the unit.

What to Expect from Your Hearing Aid

Hearing aids have tremendous capabilities, but it's unrealistic to think that a hearing aid will cure or reverse your hearing loss. A hearing aid can help you hear speech and better understand it, but it may not completely eliminate the need to ask someone to repeat a word occasionally. Talking to someone in a noisy setting still may be a little challenging.

Even if you are an experienced hearing aid user who is stepping up to a programmable hearing aid after years with a conventional model, don't expect listening perfection. These newer hearing aids offer greater clarity and quality of sound, but they can't recoup what you have already lost.

Hearing aids also don't amplify every nuance of sound. They work best when you are three to six feet from a speaker, but they are capable of picking up sounds to a distance of 10 to 15 feet. With this in mind, try to sit as close as possible to any speaker you want to hear.

As you become accustomed to deftly adjusting the volume control, and learn to better manage background noise, you will notice the difference—and you'll be using your hearing aid successfully.

DOS AND DON'TS OF HEARING AID CARE

Hearing aids work long hours and are subject to a great deal of exposure to humidity, perspiration, earwax, and the skin's natural oils. Although most manufacturers provide one-to-two-year warranties on their hearing aids, with proper care a hearing aid can last five to seven years.

Caring for your hearing aid is not a complicated process, but the device does require careful handling. Your dispenser will explain how to protect your hearing aid from adverse conditions that could damage the instrument. The basic points to remember are:

Dos

- Wipe the exterior of your hearing aid or earmold with a soft cloth or a tissue every day. This helps prevent skin oils, earwax, and perspiration from accumulating.
- Inspect your hearing aid or earmold regularly for a buildup of debris in the holes. Ask your dispenser if a specific cleaning device should be used. If you find that your hearing aid has become plugged with debris, don't attempt to remove this material yourself. Take the hearing aid to your dispenser for a cleaning.
- Disconnect the earmold from the hearing aid and wash the earmold with soap and water. *(Never place your hearing aid in water.)* A pipe cleaner can be used to dislodge any debris inside the earmold. When you have finished cleaning it, rinse it off, taking care to shake out any water inside. Allow the earmold to dry before reattaching it to your hearing aid.
- Make follow-up visits to your dispenser for regular maintenance checks and cleaning. Routine maintenance will help to keep your hearing aid in good working order.

Don'ts

- Don't allow your hearing aid to drop onto a hard surface. Its delicate inner workings may stop or malfunction. Never use alcohol or any kind of cleaning fluid to clean your hearing aid or earmold.
- Don't wear your hearing aid while showering or bathing. In fact, don't leave it in the bathroom if you are bathing—steam from the hot water may damage it. If you are washing your hair or having your hair colored, permed, or straightened, always remove the aid so that none of the chemicals can enter the instrument.
- Don't apply hairspray when you are wearing your hearing aid. It not only makes the controls and the exterior sticky, but it may gum up the interior as well and put the entire unit out of service.
- Don't keep your hearing aid in your ear if you are sweating heavily during manual labor, gardening work, or exercise. Perspiration contains salts that can work their way inside the device and cause corrosion.

- Don't expose your hearing aid to intense heat. Avoid placing it in direct sunshine, on top of a radiator, in a car's glove compartment, or any other place that can become very hot.
- Don't leave the battery inside if you won't be using the hearing aid for a long period of time. If the battery leaks, it can corrode the hearing aid.
- Don't allow children or pets access to your hearing aid. Pets especially might be tempted to gnaw on it. Bringing a chewed-up hearing aid back to your dispenser may void your warranty and you may have to pay for the repair yourself.
- Don't ever take your hearing aid apart with the intention of fixing it. This can cause the cancellation of your warranty.

Small Repairs, Major Repairs

However meticulous you are in your handling of a hearing aid, there is still a chance that it can malfunction.

Sometimes, a problem may be simple—a battery that was installed upside down, or a switch that is in the wrong position—and you can correct it yourself. If the problem calls for more expertise, your dispenser may be able to do some minor repairs in the shop. If not, the unit will have to be sent back to the manufacturer for repairs.

Every new hearing aid sold in the United States is supposed to come with at least a one-year warranty. Most manufacturers offer an extended warranty that covers repairs at an extra charge. In some cases, this warranty extension covers replacement for a lost hearing aid as well.

During the warranty extension, the manufacturer will take care of most technical or mechanical problems at no charge. If your earmold needs to be remade during this period, this work also will be covered.

If you mistreat your hearing aid and bring it back for repairs during the warranty period, the manufacturer has the right to cancel the warranty or to charge you for repairs that normally would be free. Mistreatment or abuse covers such things as dropping and smashing the hearing aid into small pieces, repairing it yourself, allowing a pet to chew on the device, or exposing it to excessive heat or moisture.

HEARING AIDS: A LOOK TO THE FUTURE

When one's hearing has become damaged, even the most advanced hearing aid cannot completely restore the ability to hear normally.

New technology, however, is making a difference in the way a hearing aid can compensate for hearing loss.

One new approach for mild hearing loss is a plastic resonating bubble that is molded and tuned for each ear. This instrument, which uses no batteries, costs less than half the price of a conventional hearing aid. It has been on the market since the late 1980s, but it is effective only for individuals with very mild hearing loss.

Current indicators point to digital technology as the wave of the future in hearing aids. The drive toward miniaturization of the components and further refinement of the technology should eventually result in smaller, more flexible hearing aids that can be better adjusted to an individual's hearing loss.

The consumer who buys today's new technology in hearing aids can expect to pay much higher prices, and this is unlikely to change in the future. As the size of the components decreases, the price will probably remain high but may be worth the investment if you can afford it.

Despite important advances, the fitting of a hearing aid by a dispenser is less than exact. As new prescriptive formulas for fitting hearing aids emerge, dispensers should be able to more scientifically fit a hearing aid to the individual.

In the past, theorists have talked about implantable hearing aids. But instead of surgically implanting a hearing aid in the middle ear, researchers have come up with hearing aids that sit very deep in the ear canal, where they can deliver more performance with less power. Time will tell which is better.

Looking very far into the future, scientists are discussing the possibility of using the body's own heat as the source of power for a hearing aid.

Hearing aids will become "smarter," as research into how human beings hear and interpret sound continues. Only by first fully understanding sound and communication can researchers then go on to make smaller and more effective hearing devices.

5

Surgical Treatments and Implants

Not every hearing-impaired person needs a hearing aid. Certain conditions that cause hearing loss can be effectively treated by surgery. Modern microsurgery and the development of new materials and devices serving as auditory replacement parts have given new hope and a better quality of life to many hard-of-hearing and deaf people.

Surgical procedures are available today to correct both cosmetic defects and hearing impairments in children born with congenital deformities of the outer ear and middle ear. Surgery may also be the treatment of choice for repairing a hole in the eardrum, helping the ear to drain properly, or for replacing diseased or damaged bone in the middle ear. Laser surgery has been especially helpful to otolaryngologists, who use it for cutting through bone and for removing scar tissue.

SURGICAL TREATMENT FOR HEARING LOSS

Your doctor may recommend surgery if your hearing loss cannot be treated effectively by medication or by other means. The most common types of surgery for hearing problems are:

- *Stapedectomy*. One of the most successful surgeries to restore hearing is a stapedectomy—the replacement of the stapes, the smallest bone in the middle ear. This surgery corrects the bone disorder known as otosclerosis (see chapter 2).
- *Tympanoplasty*. A hole in the eardrum may be patched or rebuilt. An otolaryngologist does this by removing some of the nearby muscle lining (temporalis fascia), then using this thick, taut membranous lining to repair or reconstruct the eardrum (see chapter 2).
- *Myringotomy*. This kind of surgery offers relief to children (and some adults) who suffer recurrent ear infections or persistent fluid in the middle ear, which can lead to hearing loss. In a short and simple outpatient procedure, an otolaryngologist makes a small incision in the eardrum and inserts a tiny ventilation tube. The tube promotes drainage of fluid from the middle ear and keeps it from recurring. The procedure also usually results in a marked reduction in the number and severity of ear infections.

  By inserting a ventilation tube, the surgeon is placing an artificial eustachian tube in the child's ear to allow the fluid to drain and air to flow behind the eardrum. Depending upon the type of tube used, it may stay in place for six to 18 months—until the child's own eustachian tube begins to operate properly.

  Ventilation tubes are not automatically prescribed when a child develops a middle-ear infection. The first-line treatment is still antibiotics. But when the condition fails to clear up and a child constantly shows signs of infection or hearing loss despite medication, then a ventilation tube should be considered.
- *Reconstructive surgery for congenital abnormalities*. Children who are born with incompletely developed ears (atresia) may require surgery to correct the problem. If their abnormality is due to a malformation of the eardrum, ear canal, or ossicles—all problems of the middle ear that can cause hearing loss—an otolaryngologist may be able to perform surgical reconstruction of these components to improve hearing.

  When atresia affects the external ear canal, surgery often can correct the problem as well. But atresia of the inner ear can produce a sensorineural hearing loss or progressive hearing loss that is not surgically correctable (see chapter 2).

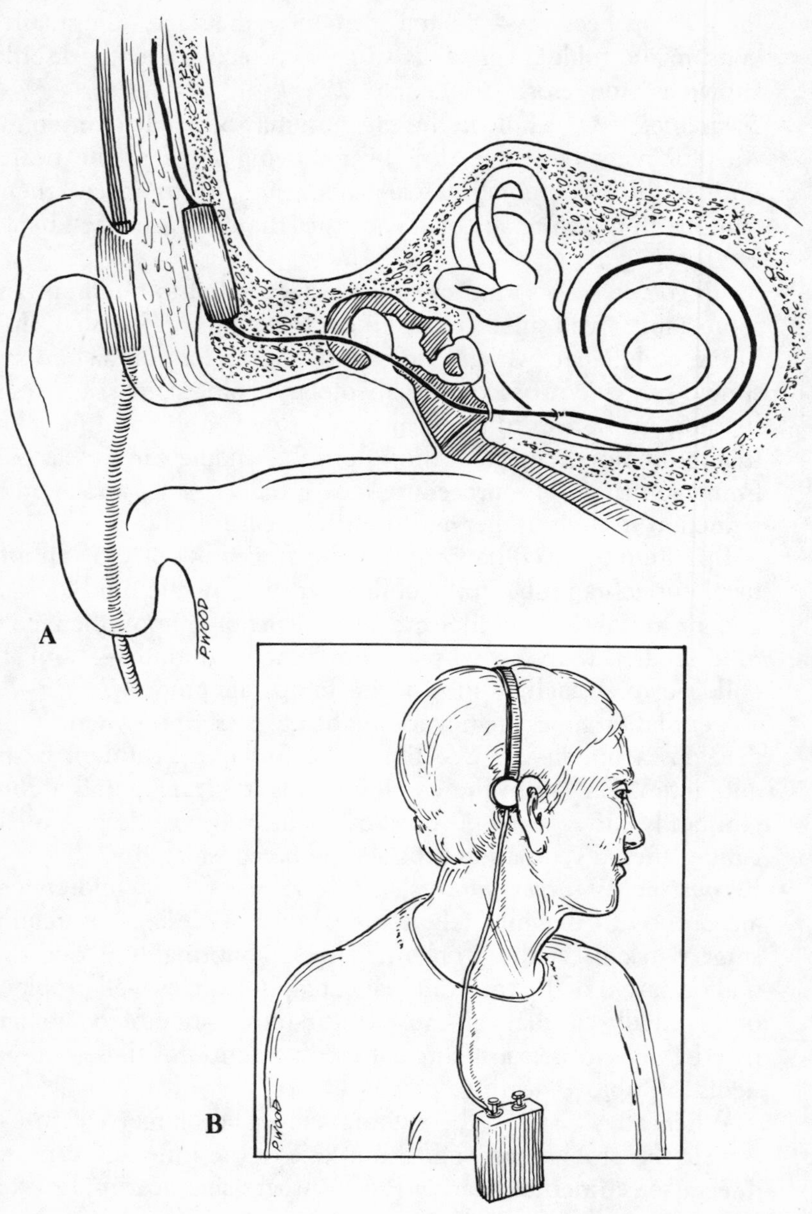

Cochlear implant: (A) inside the ear, (B) outside the ear

COCHLEAR IMPLANTS

Cochlear implants, electronic devices that are surgically implanted in the inner ear, can help bring the experience of sound to many people who are profoundly deaf. Many of those who have gained little or no benefit from a hearing aid have had significant improvements after receiving a cochlear implant.

The cochlea is the snail-shaped structure of the inner ear where sound wave vibrations are transformed into electrical nerve impulses that the brain perceives as sound. A cochlear implant bypasses the nonworking sensory hair cells that line this spiral chamber.

Although cochlear implants were first developed in the 1960s, they did not come into widespread use until the mid-1980s. They are now approved by the FDA for use in adults and children over two years of age who are either born deaf or have developed deafness after birth. As of this writing, approximately 4,800 adults and 2,000 children in the United States have received cochlear implants.

A variety of these electronic implants are now available. Each device has both internal components that are surgically implanted in the cochlea of the inner ear and external components that are worn or carried by the user.

These components include a microphone, a speech (signal) processor that functions as a minicomputer, a transmitter and receiver (signal coupler), and one or more electrodes implanted in the inner-ear area. The electrodes provide the electrical stimulation to excite the sensory cells of the cochlea, which in turn stimulate the auditory nerve.

Originally, only single-channel implants that stimulated one location in the cochlea were available. Now hearing-impaired individuals who may benefit from this type of implant can obtain multiple-channel devices that stimulate different parts of the cochlear region.

How the Implant Works

A cochlear implant delivers sound as follows: A microphone, worn behind the ear, picks up sounds that are sent through a thin cord to a small box called a signal or speech processor. (The processor itself can be worn or carried.) The processing box breaks down speech into its fundamental, useful parts and amplifies, filters, and digitizes these signals. The signal processor then selects and codes those sounds that are useful in the understanding of speech. The electronic codes are sent back up through the thin cord to the transmitter coil located behind the ear. It then sends the codes across the skin to an implanted receiver in the ear. The receiver converts these codes to electrical impulses and sends them along to the electrodes that were surgically implanted in the cochlea to stimulate the auditory nerve. The brain then recognizes these signals or codes as sound.

As perceived by the implant recipient, these sounds don't necessarily sound the same as normal speech. Rather, they may be electrical variations of familiar sounds and need to be "translated" by the hearing-impaired person.

Some implant users can detect speech and maintain normal conversations while wearing this device. Others have to learn to associate the sounds they hear with different aspects of the environment, such as traffic noises, running water, and a ringing doorbell or telephone. For many people with cochlear implants, the sounds and rhythms they receive through this device serve as important clues in learning speechreading, or lipreading. Implant recipients who get the best results are those who show an improvement in their understanding (discrimination) of speech. They may be able to understand words or sentences without having to rely solely on speechreading.

Candidates for Cochlear Implants

Studies of children who either were born deaf or became deaf before learning language have shown that cochlear implants may be valuable in helping children comprehend speech.

The ideal candidate for a cochlear implant, however, has typically been an adult or child with normal speech who once had normal hearing but has lost the ability to hear in both ears. Obviously, a child who becomes deaf after learning how to speak tends to understand speech much more rapidly than a youngster who is born deaf.

Children who lost their hearing from infections such as meningitis and then received a cochlear implant have been reported to show a rapid understanding of speech within the first six months of implantation. Small children who were deaf at birth or who became progressively deaf very early in life take much longer to understand a limited amount of speech.

Despite the success of implants in some people and promising results in others, cochlear implants are a subject of controversy in the deaf community. There are various reasons for these objections to the latest form of aural technology. One major reason is that many members of the deaf community feel that deafness is not a handicap. Another issue is a strong belief by more militant deaf people that those who haven't been able to hear from birth should learn to live with their deafness and use the traditional aids of the deaf—namely, speechreading and signing (the use of sign language).

Costs and Other Considerations

A cochlear implant is a far more expensive treatment than a hearing aid. The total cost of an implant—which includes the implant itself, a detailed evaluation as well as preoperative testing, surgery, and extensive training sessions to learn how to use the device—can range from $25,000 to $50,000.

If the specific implant device you are considering has been approved by the FDA, your health insurance company may offer benefits to cover part or all of the cost. A number of companies manufacture cochlear implant devices, and different types of devices may be under evaluation as part of a research protocol. If you or someone close to you is considering a cochlear implant, find out whether the device that will be used has been approved by the FDA, or whether it is still under investigation.

If you have decided to get a cochlear implant, it is first necessary to be accepted into an approved hospital or clinic implant program. Before acceptance, you can expect to undergo a series of evaluations, including a general physical examination, an examination of your ears, extensive hearing tests, computerized tomography (CT) scans of your inner ear, and psychological screening. The criteria used to select those who would get the best results from a cochlear implant should also be discussed.

The criteria varies from place to place, but typical requirements are

- Profound sensorineural deafness in both ears
- Inability to derive any benefit from a properly fitted hearing aid
- Deafness that was acquired after the candidate learned to use and understand speech. (If studies of young children who became deaf before learning how to talk continue to show promise, this stipulation could change.)
- Good overall physical health
- Good psychological health

Although an otolaryngologist performs cochlear implant surgery, not every ear, nose, and throat specialist is approved to perform this specialized procedure. Inquire early on if the surgeon who will be doing the procedure is approved to do this kind of work.

The Implant Procedure

The surgeon makes an incision behind the ear to open the mastoid bone. Some of the bone is removed to allow the surgical insertion of electrode wires through the middle ear and round window into the cochlea. The opposite end of the wire is attached to a receiver that is embedded in the mastoid bone and passes through the skin behind the ear.

The actual surgery may take from one and a half to five hours, depending on the type of implant used. The procedure is performed under general anesthesia, and the surgery usually requires a hospital stay of a few days.

Follow-up and Training

One to two months after surgery, you return to the health-care center for a fitting of the external parts of the device. When these components have been connected, you begin training to learn how to listen to sound through the implant.

An audiologist or another professional who specializes in the rehabilitation of the deaf prepares a training program for you. During these sessions, you learn how to associate incoming sound signals with "normal" sounds.

The degree of success you can expect to have with a cochlear implant depends on several factors. These include: your age when deafness occurred, the health of your auditory nerve, the number of years you have been deaf, your present age, and your motivation in learning how to use the device.

Certain risks accompany cochlear implant surgery, including possible complications with anesthesia, injury to the facial nerve, damage to the balance system, and infection. You must also expect the less-than-perfect hearing that results from the implant. Be certain to discuss these risks with your otolaryngologist before deciding to undergo a cochlear implant.

ALTERNATIVE TREATMENTS

An alternative to cochlear implants exists for people with no residual hearing. It is called the vibro-tactile stimulator. This device, still under study, converts acoustic signals, or sound energy, into sensations that can be felt on certain areas of the skin, such as the arms or the back.

The vibro-tactile stimulator is not an implantable device but rather one that is attached directly to the skin. Depending on whether the device picks up a high- or low-pitched sound, it alters its rhythm and the location of stimulation accordingly. The user learns to recognize the particular rhythm of incoming sounds and how to discriminate high sounds from low sounds, depending on where the device stimulates the skin.

Although a vibro-tactile stimulator does provide some information to the user, it cannot transmit sound information as rapidly as a cochlear implant can.

6

Assistive Listening Devices

The advent of computer-programmable hearing aids and cochlear implants has found many hearing-impaired people looking toward even more complex technology for help. Yet, in their quest, they may overlook a solution that already exists: assistive listening devices (ALDs).

These practical devices offer an alternative approach that can be used instead of (or with) a hearing aid for difficult listening situations. Some problem settings that typically call for improved quality of sound include a noisy restaurant, business conference, telephone conversation, lecture, sermon, or theatrical performance where background noise or distance from a speaker causes interference.

Assistive listening devices and systems can help provide the missing link between the sound source and the listener's ears. By improving the signal-to-noise ratio, these devices make the speaker's voice (the signal) louder than the noise in the immediate environment. An ALD accomplishes this because its microphone is always close to the source of sound. A hearing aid, however, cannot bridge this gap because its microphone sits in the ear, where it often picks up the speech you want to hear along with unwelcome background noise.

Although hundreds of assistive listening devices are available, they can be broken down into a few basic groups: ALDs for telephone use, for room listening, and for alerting or signaling you that someone is knocking at the door, the baby is crying, it's time to wake up, or the smoke detector has been activated.

Some ALDs cost much less than a hearing aid and can have a surprisingly pleasant effect on hearing-impaired users and the people in their lives. Despite the availability of these products, however, their use by people with hearing impairments has been slow to catch on.

Many users of these devices admit to being skeptical and uninterested at first, but they change their minds after trying them. The reasons for acceptance: better reception of sound without background noise from a sound amplifier, and better ability to hear a speaker who is more than three feet away.

How to Buy an ALD

A growing array of assistive listening devices—many of them with improved technology—are now on the market. Some manufacturers, nonprofit organizations, and schools have demonstration centers nationwide where you can visit and examine these products. For those who can't easily travel, many of these centers also have ALD catalogs that can be ordered by mail.

Buying an ALD is not like buying a toaster or a hair dryer. Choosing an assistive listening device often calls for additional guidance. For that reason, it is wise to consult an otologist, otolaryngologist, or audiologist for recommendations on purchasing the most appropriate one for your needs.

Unfortunately, there is currently no central source of information on assistive listening technology for hearing professionals or consumers. Some demonstration centers have trained knowledgeable staff who not only can explain how to use the various products, but are also willing to review the benefits and limitations of each one. Other centers may operate as storefront franchises that sell only a small number of ALDs.

In addition to demonstration centers, some retail and electronics stores may carry some of these products, and others are available through catalogs or directly from the manufacturer. For a list of ALD demonstration centers, contact the National Information Center on Deafness or the nonprofit Self-Help for Hard-of-Hearing People (see appendix C).

For a special review of devices that were evaluated exclusively for this book by the technical staff of *Consumer Reports* magazine, see appendix B.

Visiting a Demonstration Center

If you are interested in assistive listening devices and are within driving distance of a demonstration center, you may want to visit the center to view or buy some of these products. It's wise to call first to find out the hours of the center and whether you need an appointment. Some places may prefer to set aside a block of time to show you the products and demonstrate how they work.

When you call, ask the representative some questions:

- Is an appointment necessary?
- Will you perform a hands-on demonstration?
- Do you sell products as well as offer demonstrations?
- Do you have a qualified staff member who can provide the appropriate training to operate the devices for sale?
- Does the center mainly serve as a dispenser of assistive devices?
- If I am undecided about buying an item, can I lease it instead?
- What is your policy regarding returns? Do you have a trial period with purchases?

TYPES OF ASSISTIVE LISTENING DEVICES: TELEPHONE-RELATED ALDS

Assistive devices for the telephone range from simple amplifiers for a mild-to-moderate hearing loss to sophisticated communication devices with computerized memory for those who are profoundly deaf.

Telephone Amplifiers

Telephone amplifiers are geared toward people with varying degrees of hearing loss. An amplifier allows you to increase the loudness of the incoming sound on your telephone by adjusting a volume control switch. These devices are fairly simple to operate, and they can be used for:

- *Public telephones*. Perhaps the simplest and most recognizable amplifying device is the one found on public telephones in many locations. (A telephone that is equipped to amplify the incoming conversation is indicated by a recognizable symbol.) To operate the amplifier, you just push a button to make the incoming sound louder.
- *Portable units*. Portable amplifiers are available that can be strapped onto any phone. These battery-powered units are small enough to carry around in your pocket or purse, and offer a simple solution if you are a frequent phone user—especially when away from home or work. Some portable amplifiers may not be compatible with all phones.
- *Amplified handsets*. An amplified handset is another home phone option. Before you buy one, you may want to check to see that it can be attached to standard older styles as well as modern telephones. These units usually feature a volume control setting. Some may get their power from the phone line while others require a battery.
- *In-line amplifiers*. These amplifiers plug into the telephone between the handset and the base of the phone. A volume control on the small amplifier box allows you to increase or lower the volume. Not all in-line amplifiers are compatible with all telephones.
- *Telecoil*. If you wear a hearing aid that has telecoil circuitry, you can use your T-coil to hear a telephone conversation more effectively. When this switch is turned on, it picks up and amplifies electromagnetic voice signals from the telephone receiver instead of amplifying sound waves. All public telephones and those that are sold for consumer use now must be compatible with telecoil circuitry (see chapter 4).

  A hearing aid equipped with a T-coil also enables you to use the aid to hear more clearly in a large listening area that is equipped with an audio loop, FM system, or infrared system. An FM system, however, only works if you have a neckloop, or if the room is equipped with an audio loop system.

Telecommunications Devices

Profoundly deaf individuals and those people who are in regular contact with hearing-impaired relatives, friends, and associates usually

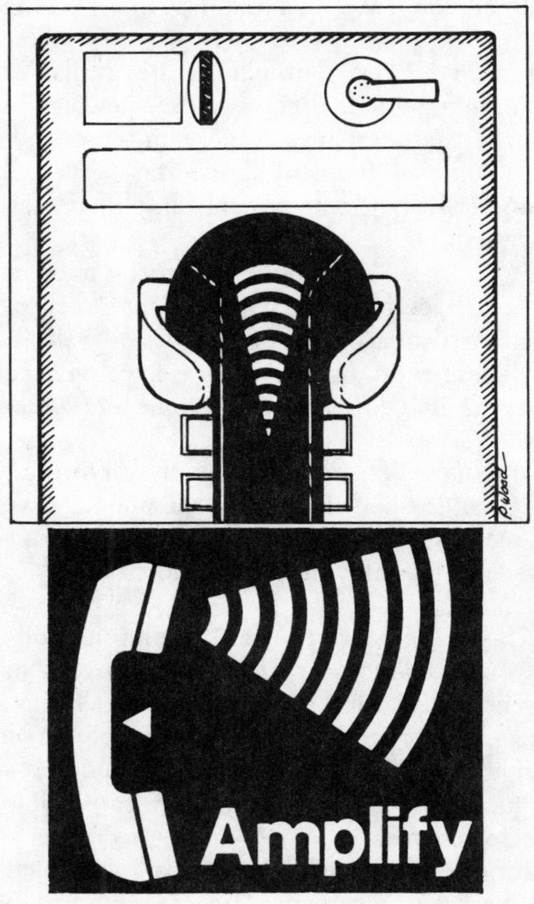

Public telephone amplification symbols

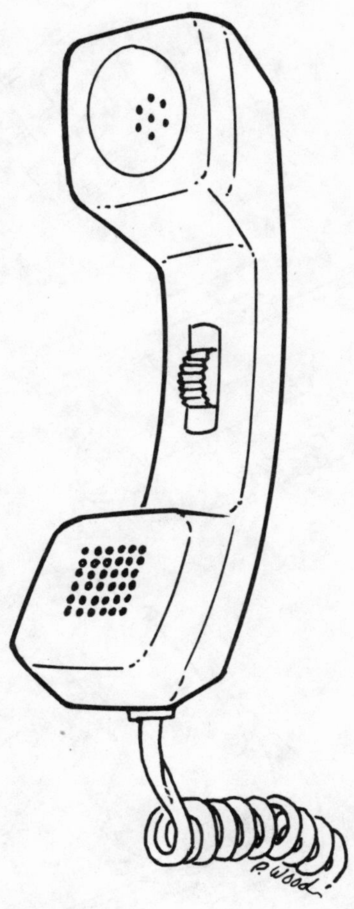

Amplified telephone handset with volume control

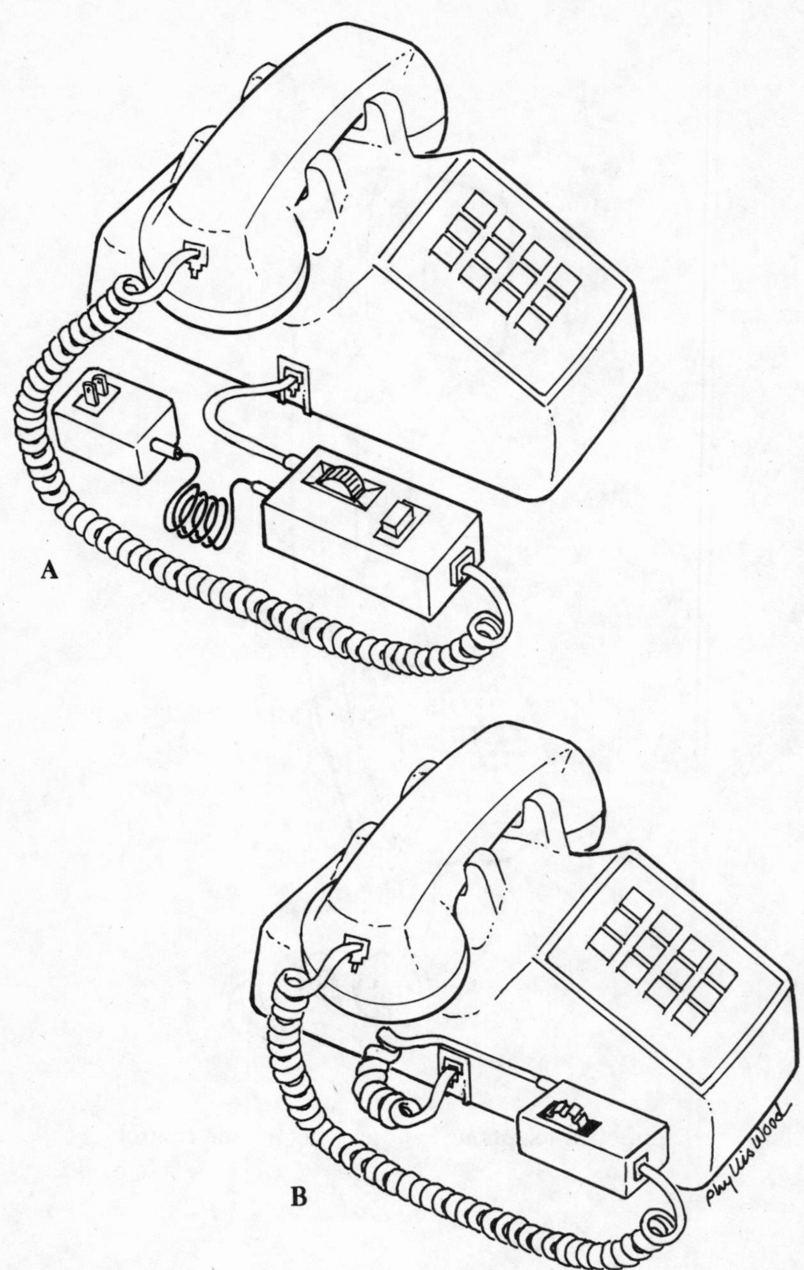

(A) Transformer-powered in-line telephone amplifier
(B) Line-powered in-line amplifier

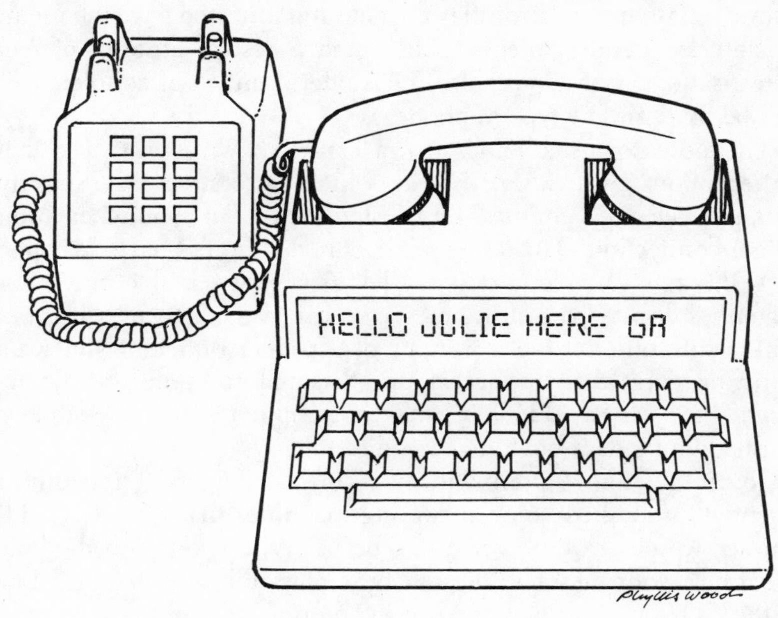

Telecommunications device for the deaf (TDD or TTY)

find *telecommunications devices for the deaf (TDDs)* to be highly useful. These products can send typewritten messages over the telephone, eliminating any need for voice contact.

TDD is a term that is often used interchangeably with TTY, an acronym that stands for the old-style teletypewriters once used by telegraph companies and newswire services. Such equipment transmitted typed information over telephone lines, and it was also received as a typed message.

A basic TDD model closely resembles the TTY typewriter keyboard, while the smaller, compact TDD models are strikingly similar to lightweight notepad computers that fold up and fit in a pocketbook, briefcase, or backpack. Once the connection is made between two people equipped with TDDs, then telecommunication can take place by means of typed messages instead of speech.

Features. Some of the newer TDDs offer a two-line display of the text as it is being transmitted, a backlit screen, and a long-lasting battery pack. Certain units also display the date and time and have the memory to store frequently called numbers and a certain amount of recent conversations. Some portable TDDs offer a universal coupler, which can be used for any type of phone.

The more expensive TDDs have a feature known as enhanced acoustic reception sensitivity, or EARS, which can increase the sensitivity of the device and help the TDD "listen harder," a boon when you get a poor connection. The less expensive models do not have this option.

TDDs are available in desk models as well as portable units. Some machines display part of the message on a visual screen as it is being sent, while others have a printer, or a printer outlet, if you want a printed record of the conversation. Personal computers also can be adapted to serve as a TDD. To make a computer TDD-accessible, you must add a modem board to the unit.

Some TDDs have automatic answering capabilities. These units are essentially modified voice answering machines that record the TDD sounds, which are simply acoustic beeps. When you push the button to retrieve your message, the machine plays the recorded beeps back to the TDD and the message is printed out. Some of these answering machines are designed to be used for both hearing and TDD users alike.

Telephone relay service. More public phones are beginning to be TDD-equipped. Another variation on TDD use is the *telephone relay service*. This service has been offered in some states in the past but is now required in all states as a provision of the Americans with Disabilities Act of 1990.

Someone who is deaf can call a hearing person—one without a TDD—by calling a relay operator. It works this way: The caller types in the relay operator's number, then the phone number of the person to be contacted, and the message. The relay operator calls the desired number and reads the message to the hearing person. If that person responds, the operator types this message and relays it back to the original caller.

All calls are kept confidential, and the operator does not keep records of the calls. Only billing records are kept so that the call can be charged to the correct telephone account number.

ROOM LISTENING DEVICES

Various methods are available for enhancing audio signals for group listening in large rooms, or for individual listening situations such as watching television at home.

The key to successful listening with these systems is the placement of the microphone. By positioning the mike no more than six inches from the speaker's mouth, the sound comes in without interference from echoes, reverberations, or background noise. Among these products are audio loops, FM systems, infrared systems, and hard-wired devices.

Audio Loops

An audio loop system is made up of a microphone and an amplifier attached to a length of wire that encircles, or loops, around the area where enhanced sound is needed.

The electric current that flows through the loop creates a magnetic field that can be picked up by hearing aid wearers inside the loop who switch on the T-coil on their hearing aids. Loop listeners without T-coils or hearing aids can also hear the enhanced sound by wearing a special portable receiver.

In some public places, including auditoriums, museums, classrooms, and houses of worship, an audio loop may be a permanent installation that is connected to the public-address system. Loop systems are also available for smaller groups of people, such as in a conference room. If the room is fairly small and quiet, the microphone could be placed in the center of the table to enhance the voices of each person who speaks during the meeting.

A personal induction loop device can also be purchased for use in the home. The long, thin wire that comes with these units is easily placed under a rug or around the molding in a room. The wire is then attached to a transmitter, which is hooked to a microphone or an audio input, such as a television set.

Disadvantages. While a loop system is easy to install and highly practical for people who already use a hearing aid, there are problems with its use. For example, the magnetic field created in the loop is susceptible to interference from other similar electromagnetic fields and signals. And if the telecoil in your hearing aid isn't very powerful or is poorly positioned, this may affect the results. The strength of the signal within the looped area also may vary in different parts of the loop.

FM Systems

FM (frequency modulation) systems use transmitters to broadcast sound exactly the same way as does a radio station. The sound or speech is carried from the FM microphone to a small FM receiver that is worn by the listener.

An antenna is built into the cord of the headphones to assist in picking up the transmission. Each transmission is assigned an actual channel number and a frequency designation, just as if it were a radio station broadcast.

The frequencies that have been allocated primarily for hearing-impaired listeners are in the 72-to-76-megahertz band—numbers that you won't find on your radio dial. With the growing use of cellular phones and mobile paging systems, however, it's not unusual for FM-system users to get interference from these other forms of communication.

An FM system that's working normally can deliver high-quality sound with reduced interference. Just as with an audio loop, the speaker's voice must be no more than six inches from the microphone for the listener to get the best sound reception. If the speaker strays from the microphone, however, the hearing-impaired person cannot hear the words. With this problem in mind, some facilities have installed base station transmitters that pick up the speaker's voice in the same fashion as the smaller microphones. The difference is that this setup is hooked into the room's existing public address system.

Hooking in to FM. FM systems can be used to deliver sound in various ways, including direct audio input, a T-coil on a hearing aid, neckloops, and silhouette coils.

- *Direct audio input*. When a hearing aid has a direct audio input option, the transmission—or output—from the FM receiver can be connected by a cord directly to the aid. If you intend to use your hearing aid in conjunction with the receiver of an FM system, be certain that you buy a cord with the proper specifications.

- *Neckloops.* A neckloop, a wire worn around the neck, can take sound and convert it into magnetic energy. This is a worthwhile option if you have a T-coil on your hearing aid and the speaker is using a microphone that sends the sound directly to your neckloop. It works like an audio loop system, only on an individual basis.
- *Silhouette coils.* A silhouette coil or inductor is another method of hooking an FM system to a hearing aid. This device, which can be used instead of a neckloop, also delivers sound through a magnetic field. The coil looks like a flat behind-the-ear hearing aid and fits right next to your own aid when it is in use. To operate a silhouette coil, the hearing aid's telecoil must be in the "T" position.

Flexibility of FM systems. An FM system offers more flexibility than an audio loop because the transmission can be sent over a wider area. Because the sound is transmitted via radio waves, the system doesn't need wires.

Originally, FM systems were used only in classrooms for hearing-impaired students. In an educational setting, they are called FM auditory training systems. Personal FM systems—or those that are designed to be used with a personal hearing aid in some way—have evolved from these auditory trainers. Many large listening facilities now offer FM systems for hearing-impaired people.

Some theaters or large concert halls have FM receivers available for rent, and many theater managers say it is not unusual for a hearing-impaired person to call the theater in advance and ask which frequency the theater's FM system uses. These theatergoers are likely to bring their own FM receivers or neckloops to wear during the performance.

Disadvantages. One limitation of an FM system is the potential for interference from another transmission in the same listening area. Another concern is privacy. Occasionally, an FM transmission may be received outside the area for which it is intended.

Infrared Systems

Infrared listening systems are common today in theaters, movies, auditoriums, and houses of worship. They usually are free but require a deposit that is refundable when the unit is returned. An infrared

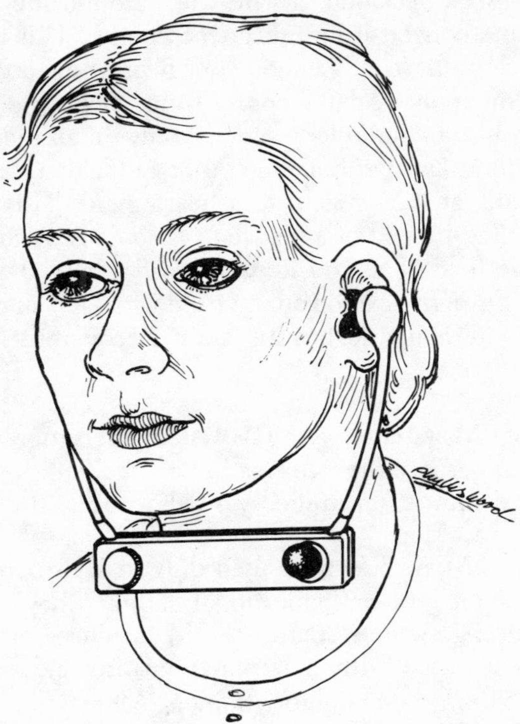

Under-the-chin headset receiver and transmitter

system converts sound to harmless, invisible, infrared light waves that are turned back into sound again by a receiver worn by the listener.

When an infrared system is needed for a large listening area, the institution will contact a company that specializes in these products. Finally, an electrician must be called in to properly install the system so that all infrared users in the room can have access to the sound transmission.

Infrared systems are also available for the home and other small-room listening needs. Typically, this kind of system uses a portable transmitter that plugs into any outlet. The microphone can be attached to the front of the speaker on your television set. Or, if someone in the room wanted to carry on a conversation with you, he or she could just talk into the microphone and you would receive the amplified voice sounds through your receiver.

Infrared receivers can be hooked into a headset, a hearing aid, or a neckloop. All infrared receivers make use of a diode—a tiny transparent dome that catches the infrared light waves for transmission to your ears.

If you have a mild-to-moderate hearing loss and don't wear a hearing aid, you can use a headset receiver that hooks right onto your ears. This kind of headset, which is called an under-the-chin set, has a volume control dial and a diode that is sensitive to the infrared light. Some headsets may be more powerful or more comfortable than others, so shop around for the right one for you.

If you do wear a hearing aid, you can connect the infrared receiver directly to the aid. If the hearing aid has a T-coil, switch it into the "T" position and the receiver can be connected to a neckloop or a silhouette coil.

All personal infrared receivers are compatible with the systems used in large listening areas. Many people who use them at home may bring their own headset receivers along to theaters or auditoriums, if they so choose.

Disadvantages. An infrared system cannot be used outdoors or in a room that is filled with natural light. This is because the sun's light contains high levels of infrared light. Normally, an infrared receiver is free of static, but interference from sunlight or daylight can cause the device to make buzzing sounds.

Another limitation of infrared systems is that the wearer must face the transmitter directly in order to receive the signal clearly.

Hard-Wired Devices

Hard-wired devices are actually connected by wire to the source of the sound—unlike the wireless FM and infrared systems. They deliver sound directly from a speaker wearing a microphone or from a television set to the listener.

These simple and compact amplifying units are similar to body hearing aids. They employ a small amplifier that must be carried or worn in a pocket or clipped onto a belt. People who use hearing aids, as well as those who don't, have found this device useful in a variety of settings: in restaurants, in the car, at home or at work, and while watching TV.

Many users find that these units offer a high-quality signal and improve the quality of speech over background noise well enough to allow them to enjoy television or carry on a one-to-one conversation. In some cases, people who have had poor results with a hearing aid find that these devices work better for them.

You can use them with a TV set or a radio, and can adjust the sound as needed without increasing the volume to levels that would disturb other listeners.

These units are less expensive than hearing aids. Accessories are available, including a neckloop if you have a hearing aid with a T-coil, headphones, and rechargeable batteries.

Disadvantages. Although personal hearing units offer quality sound, they have their limitations, too. A main problem is restricted mobility—it may be inconvenient or difficult to make a wired connection in some circumstances. And the device is not practical for use in a large listening area.

ALERTING AND SIGNALING DEVICES

Ingenious attention-getters are among the many alerting devices available for people with a hearing impairment. Such sounds as a ringing doorbell, a telephone, or a blaring smoke alarm have been adapted into effective alerting and signaling devices.

The theory behind these products is that different visual or tactile signals can effectively substitute for a signal that is heard only by those with normal hearing.

Different devices exist for various situations. Among them are a smoke alarm that triggers a flashing strobe light and a powerful bed shaker that wakes a sleeping person. Another is a receiver that allows a hearing-impaired listener to know when the baby is crying or the doorbell is ringing—the pattern of the flashing from a lamp or special light differs in each case.

Certain alerting devices are designed to be used in one area only, whereas others can be plugged into remote receivers in other rooms around the home. One consideration is that the remote receivers work with the alerting device only when they share a common electrical circuit. Check the electrical hookups of certain rooms of your house by looking at the diagram inside your circuit box. Apartment dwellers may have to go from room to room, plugging in the unit and figuring out on their own which rooms have a common circuit.

All of these signaling devices can be bought separately. Some are available as an overall system that monitors the telephone, baby's crib, doorbell, and smoke alarm.

CLOSED CAPTIONING

Television viewers who find it difficult to understand speech on TV—even while using one of the room listening systems—may find tele-captions extremely helpful.

Many television programs are captioned for hearing-impaired listeners, but the printed data can be seen only on television sets equipped with a decoder. This system of telecaptions is called *closed captioning*. To indicate which programs have captions, television listings commonly use the letters "CC." (Videotapes with captions also carry the same mark.) Federal law now requires all new televisions to have built-in decoder circuitry that can be switched on or off at will.

In the past, captions were presented in white letters on a black background. Now, some manufacturers are offering captions in color. If you are planning to buy a new TV set, check to make sure that the set you are purchasing includes a built-in decoder.

This new circuitry will eventually make telecaption decoders obsolete. In the meantime, assistive listening device sales centers and electronics stores are likely to have some of these units available or at least will know which manufacturers still plan to produce them.

The Americans with Disabilities Act does not require that program producers provide captions for every program, but about 175 hours of television programs are now closed-captioned every week. Practically all of the major networks' prime-time offerings are captioned.

7

How to Prevent Hearing Loss

Physicians and other health-care professionals have learned how to prevent much of the infection-related deafness that once affected newborns and to treat other medical problems that can lead to a loss of hearing. But a more alarming menace is increasingly disturbing and endangering our hearing: noise.

Unfortunately, warnings about protecting ourselves from noise have fallen too often on deaf ears. Estimates by the National Institutes of Health say that about 10 million people in the United States have already suffered permanent hearing loss from exposure to excessive noise, whether in the workplace, off the job, or at home.

PROTECTING YOUR EARS AT WORK

Noise is a leading occupational hazard. Some of the noisiest jobs are those in mining, manufacturing, lumber, metalworking, agriculture, drilling, and construction. People who work around noisy equipment or who are exposed to especially loud explosions of sound are also at high risk.

The federal government, in the form of the Occupational Safety and Health Administration (OSHA), regulates noise in the workplace. The agency's current noise standard allows a worker to be exposed to 90 decibels of constant noise over an eight-hour period. This standard is five decibels higher than the level advocated by the Environmental Protection Agency, which prefers a standard of 85 decibels for an eight-hour shift.

A five-decibel difference may not seem that significant, but hearing experts agree that the higher level of noise represented by the extra five decibels can produce permanent hearing loss after a number of years of such exposure. Another problem with the OSHA standard is that it represents an average and doesn't protect everyone, since some people are very sensitive to noise while others are more resistant to its harmful effects.

OSHA bases its standard on what is called a "time-weighted average." When the noise level in a work area exceeds 90 decibels, workers can still be exposed to the noise—but for a shorter period of time. With each five-decibel increase in noise, the time a worker is allowed to remain in that area is reduced by half.

OSHA Noise Standards

90 decibels—eight hours of exposure a day
95 decibels—four hours of exposure a day
100 decibels—two hours of exposure a day
115 decibels—15 minutes of exposure a day

Since the adoption of noise standards for all U.S. employees in 1971, OSHA has required that industries place controls on machinery to mitigate some of the noise produced on the job. The demise of the federal noise abatement program in 1982, however, has weakened enforcement of these standards. OSHA remains responsible for enforcing federal noise regulations, but the number of citations issued to employers for ineffective noise-reduction controls has dropped considerably over the last decade.

In place of routine inspections, OSHA has allowed many employers to participate in its voluntary protection program to prevent and control occupational hazards, including noise. Employers with voluntary programs designate an employee to serve as a contact person with OSHA.

If any safety or health problems arise that cannot be resolved at the workplace, the employee representative must contact the agency. The rationale behind this program is to free up OSHA's inspectors to visit establishments that are less likely to comply with standards.

OSHA also requires that some companies provide hearing advice and guidance for their workers.

Industrial Hearing-Conservation Programs

Companies with work areas where the noise level surpasses the minimum standard are required by law to establish hearing-conservation programs. Each company's program must include the following requirements:

- Identifying work areas where potentially hazardous noise levels exist
- Scheduling regular hearing screening tests for employees
- Requiring and enforcing the proper wearing of personal hearing protection by employees
- Requesting management to take measures to control noise in high-noise areas
- Educating workers on the dangers of exposure to noise
- Documenting hearing test results, noise surveys, education programs, and plant inspections
- Making sure a worker with damaged hearing has the appropriate care to ensure that there is no further hearing loss

Even when companies provide an effective hearing-conservation program and diligently enforce it, it has been estimated that only 90 percent of the exposed workers will be protected from noise-induced hearing loss. Unfortunately, there is no way of knowing in advance whether one individual is more vulnerable to noise injury than another. Periodic screening tests, however, can help identify these individuals before significant hearing loss has occurred.

The best way to reduce the risk of occupational hearing loss is to eliminate noise at its source. Ideally, a physical plant should be built with soundproof barriers or booths incorporated into its basic design. When there are no protective noise barriers, the only way to remedy the problem is by means of engineering controls.

One engineering solution that can lower noise levels in a plant includes placing sound-absorbent materials on the walls and ceilings. In other cases, a modification of a noisy machine part can help, including replacing worn-out gears and bearings or just tightening a bolt. Mounting a noisy piece of equipment on rubber padding also can result in a lower noise level. When engineering controls fail to solve the problem, or such changes are not economically feasible, then hearing protection must be worn by all workers in the area affected.

PROTECTING YOUR HEARING OFF THE JOB

Mounting evidence has shown that exposure to excessive noise during leisure hours can be hazardous. Unfortunately, many of these hours spent "relaxing" are also spent partaking in high-decibel activities, such as listening to loud live or amplified music, or by hunting and target shooting.

Live or Amplified Music

Early in the 1970s, researchers found that the decibels routinely registered in many rock concerts and discotheques hovered well above the 100 mark. Despite warnings about the potential dangers of constant exposure to excessively loud music, the bands have played on. By the early 1980s, the amplified speakers used at rock concerts typically had 20,000 to 30,000 watts of power. Today's amplifiers are equipped with 100,000 to 500,000 watts.

Studies of the effect of exposure to amplified music on the audience have shown that most people develop a moderate and temporary threshold shift in their hearing. This means that while they may lose about 30 decibels of their normal hearing ability during the concert, they usually recover normal hearing in a few hours or even a few days. But those who frequently attend rock concerts or always sit near the speakers may be at risk of suffering permanent hearing damage. Teenagers and young adults who expose themselves to regular doses of amplified rock music may develop cumulative damage to their hearing.

In contrast, researchers who analyzed the effect of sound levels at classical concerts came to a different conclusion. They found that although the musicians in the orchestra may develop some noise-induced hearing loss, the audience is unlikely to have a problem. This is the case even for classical music lovers who spend up to 20 hours a week at concerts. The average exposure at a classical concert is about 90 decibels.

Little information is available on levels of exposure at live jazz concerts, but one researcher who took a sound level meter to a big band concert found the average level of noise exposure was 96 decibels.

How to protect your hearing. Buy a pair of earplugs and take them with you when you go to live rock concerts or noisy clubs. You'll still be able to hear the music, but the plugs can cut the decibel level.

Walkabout Stereo Players

Many devotees of high-decibel rock and rap music prefer to keep the volume high on their walkabout stereo players. A British study of 15-to-23-year-olds concluded that those who regularly used walkabouts *and* attended rock concerts had a rate of hearing loss that was double that of young people without such exposure. Some of these walkabout stereos are capable of producing sound as loud as 126 decibels—a level equivalent to a chain saw or jackhammer.

But young people aren't the only ones at risk: Many adults who wear these units use them to block out the sounds of a noisy environment. Some even wear walkabouts while working inside a noisy factory and may be boosting their noise exposure to well above acceptable levels. In some localities, of course, it is illegal to drive or jog and wear a personal stereo player because the unit acoustically isolates the wearer from possible warning signs of danger.

How to protect your hearing. When using a walkabout, keep the volume at a reasonable level. As a rule of thumb, if someone standing next to you can hear the music coming from your headphones, the volume is too high. Follow the same advice when wearing a headset that is attached to a larger stereo unit, a video game, or a television set. Never use headphones to drown out other noise in a room. After listening for a while, take a break and give your hearing a rest.

Hunting and Target Shooting

After work-related noise, exposure to the noise of guns has become this country's most serious hearing hazard. It is estimated that more than half of American men who work in industry also fire guns occasionally. This statistic is not surprising—the National Rifle Association claims that 70 million Americans are gun owners and that 20 million buy hunting licenses each year.

Noisy Leisure-Time Activities

Music
Rock concerts
Discotheques and clubs
Personal stereo players/walkabouts
Oversized amplifiers in cars or trucks

Firearms
Hunting
Target practice
Skeet shooting

Outdoor/Indoor Sports
Motorcycles
Dirt bikes
Speedboats
Snowmobiles
Model airplanes
Racing cars
Cockpit of private planes
Enclosed sports stadiums
Video arcade games
Fireworks

Hobbies/Chores
Chain saws
Power tools
Lawn mowers
Snow blowers

Measurements with sound level meters have shown that a .22 caliber rifle can produce 132 decibels per single shot. A high-powered shotgun can fire about 172 decibels. A single round from a shotgun or a high-powered pistol or rifle contains enough acoustic energy to equal a 90-decibel exposure for a workweek of eight-hour days. One researcher has compared shooting a box of 50 shells in one session as the equivalent of spending a year working in a factory where the decibel level is constantly at 90.

Noise-induced hearing loss usually affects both ears, but because a rifle is held diagonal to the body, the ear that is closest to the butt of the gun usually suffers less damage. When a round is fired, the opposite ear is exposed to the greater noise and tends to develop a more profound hearing loss.

How to protect your hearing. Wear hearing protection when you are target shooting, skeet shooting, or hunting. Special types of earmuffs offer the best protection.

Noise Around the Home

As American households keep adding more appliances, there is growing concern about noise levels in the home. Most modern devices and appliances aren't hazardous to hearing, however, unless you use them for long periods of time.

The sound decibel levels for some typical appliances are:

Appliance	Decibels
Air conditioner	50–69
Alarm clock	64–76
Coffee maker (percolator)	54
Coffee grinder	75–80
Dishwasher	55–71
Electric shaver	48–80
Electric drill	91
Vacuum cleaner	60–85
Garbage disposal	67–93
Hair dryer	59–71
Telephone	77
Toilet flushing	76–82
Washing machine	49–72

Other higher-decibel items that consumers should be more concerned about are gasoline-powered leaf blowers and chain saws. Loudness measurements for one leaf blower recorded maximum levels of 112 decibels. When the overall amount of exposure was calculated, the average sound level was 102.6 decibels. (Daily exposure at this level for an hour and a half would violate the OSHA standard for the workplace.)

Similarly, a chain saw running at idle can produce from 91 to 98 decibels. But when used during cutting, sound levels have been reported to reach 116 decibels.

How to protect your hearing. Wear hearing protection when operating a gasoline-powered leaf blower or a chain saw. Use either earplugs or special earmuffs.

TYPES OF HEARING PROTECTION

Manufacturers of hearing-protection devices are required to provide a noise-reduction rating—or performance rating—for each one. In theory, a higher rating means that a product offers better protection. In practice, it may mean that laboratory testing conditions are very different from those found on the job.

The size of the hearing protector, as well as its design and material, has an effect on how much it can reduce the amount of incoming sound. When plugs or muffs are properly fitted, they can reduce the intensity of sound by 15 to 30 decibels. Earplugs are considered better protection against low-frequency noise, whereas earmuffs work better against high-frequency sounds. The use of earplugs and earmuffs together can add 10 to 15 additional decibels of protection. When noise levels exceed 105 decibels, it is recommended that you combine the two for better protection.

In order to be effective, the device must be worn continuously. Workers who remove their earplugs for one hour of a noisy eight-hour workday would have a significant reduction in hearing protection. Instead of getting 30 decibels of sound reduction, they would get only a reduction average of nine decibels for the day. The unprotected hour of exposure subjects workers to 1,000 times more sound energy than they would experience while wearing hearing protection.

Keep in mind that decibels are measured on a logarithmic scale.

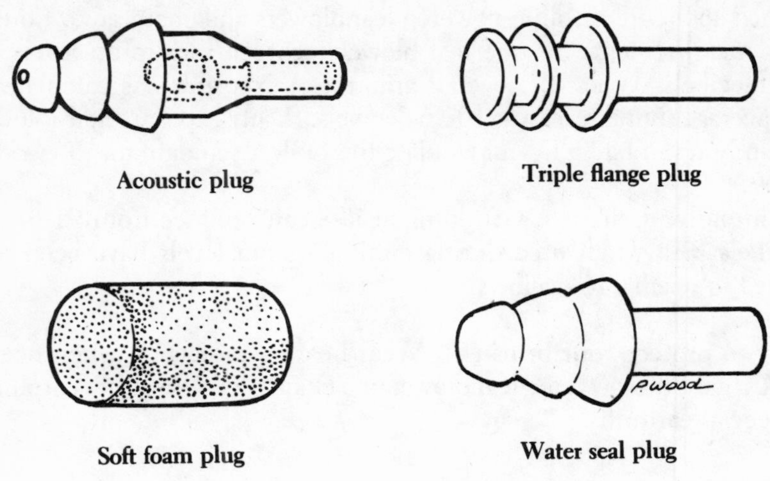

Acoustic plug

Triple flange plug

Soft foam plug

Water seal plug

Types of earplugs

Each time the sound level increases by 10 decibels, the sound energy increases by 10 times the amount of the lower figure.

Earplugs

Earplugs are light, comfortable, and easy to carry. General-purpose earplugs for jobs like mowing the lawn or using power tools are inexpensive and can be bought at pharmacies, retail outlets, and sporting goods stores.

Custom-made earplugs are available from an audiologist. A mold of your ear canal is made so that the shape of the plug matches exactly. A custom device may be more comfortable to wear, but its effectiveness is about the same as an over-the-counter earplug. Unknown to most of their audience, many classical and rock musicians wear custom-made earplugs during a performance. In order to allow the musicians to hear the higher frequencies of notes while still protecting their ears, some of these custom devices employ special features. One plug may have a built-in acoustic amplifier, while another may use special vents.

Among the materials used in earplugs are foam, acrylic, glass fiber, rubber, wax, and cotton that has been impregnated with a soft wax. Many people think a wad of cotton in the ear will dampen noise, but these homemade plugs are worthless.

No matter which type of earplug you use, it's important to get a good fit. Because many people have ear canals of different sizes, it may be necessary to wear a different size plug in each ear. If you are buying earplugs for the first time, you will have to experiment with different brands and types until you find the right fit.

Earplugs aren't difficult to use, but it's important to learn how to insert them properly. One recommended method: With your hand, reach around behind your head. Pull on the top part of your ear (the pinna) upward and outward while inserting the plug with your other hand. This movement helps the ear canal open up to receive the earplug.

Inserting an earplug rarely harms the eardrum. This is because the eardrum and deeper regions of the ear canal are especially sensitive to pressure and pain. If you come too close to these areas with an earplug, you will feel the discomfort and realize that this is a signal to stop pushing the plug in any farther.

Even when earplugs make a good seal in your ear canal, they can work themselves loose and must be reinserted. Certain activities, even chewing gum, may loosen the plugs. Certain premolded and fiberglass earplugs tend to work loose more easily than foam and custom-molded plugs.

Remove earplugs—especially premolded inserts—slowly. Check the plugs routinely for signs of shrinkage, hardening, cracking, and other indications of wear. Earplugs should retain their original shape and resiliency—otherwise they can lose their effectiveness.

Some earplugs are intended to be thrown out after a single use. Others are reusable and washable. Check the manufacturer's instructions for cleaning the earplugs.

Earmuffs

Special protective earmuffs are much more effective against high noise levels than earplugs are. Some airport workers, jackhammer operators, military personnel, and target shooters are typical wearers.

Muffs are usually attached to a band that is worn across the head, or they may be mounted into a helmet or hard hat that protects the head as well as the ears. Each of the cushioned earcups is filled with a sound-absorbent material that forms a seal around the entire ear. As long as the seal remains tight and intact, the earmuffs are effective. When communication is necessary, a one-way radio link can be incorporated into the muffs.

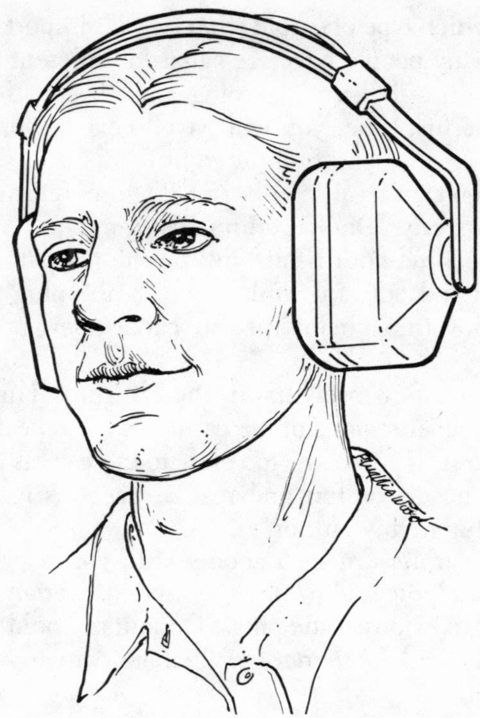

Protective earmuffs

Although muffs are easy to adjust and offer good sound protection, they can be uncomfortable when worn in hot and humid weather. They are also more expensive than earplugs.

Canal Caps

This type of hearing protection resembles earplugs. The "caps" are attached to a band that may be worn over or behind the head, or under the chin. These protectors are used mainly by workers who, for whatever reason, must repeatedly remove and replace them.

Unlike plugs and muffs, canal caps tend to feel uncomfortable if worn for too long. Some of these devices slightly enter the ear canal, while others do not. Caps that don't enter beyond the opening of the ear canal have a greater chance of losing their seal if the band is accidentally knocked ajar.

For a Quieter Home Environment

There are many steps you can take to reduce the amount of noise in your home:

- Use sound-absorbing materials such as carpeting, drapes, and upholstered furniture to help dampen noise.
- Place a foam or rubber pad under typewriters, printers, food processors, and other noisy equipment.
- When you operate power mowers, leaf blowers, and chain saws, wear hearing protection.
- Play stereo equipment, television, and radios at moderate volumes. Be considerate of your neighbors.
- Be cautious when buying toys for children. Avoid toys that make loud or explosive sounds.
- Before buying an appliance, find out its noise level. If a demonstration isn't possible, or you are ordering from a catalog, call the manufacturer to find out the decibel level of the appliance.

PREVENTING PAINFUL (TEMPORARY) HEARING LOSS

Airplane Travel

Changes in atmospheric pressure during an airplane flight may cause a particularly uncomfortable form of temporary hearing loss. If you plan to fly and you want to avoid the intense ear pain of aerotitis (barotrauma), there are various techniques that may prove helpful.

The key to maintaining comfort is to keep the pressure on the outside of both eardrums equal to the pressure inside the middle ear. Problems can occur when an insufficient amount of fresh air enters the eustachian tube, a thin tube that connects the back of the nose with the middle ear. By keeping the supply of air constant, you may be able to equalize the air pressure in your ears. When the air pressure is not equal, your ears will feel blocked.

Most travelers have heard the advice to yawn frequently, chew gum, and suck on mints or hard candy just before and during the plane's descent. All of these activities encourage swallowing and help to keep the eustachian tube open. Yawning is the best of these techniques because it moves the muscle that opens the eustachian tube more effectively.

Avoid sleeping when the airplane is descending because you may not be able to produce enough swallowing action to equalize the air pressure. (Ask the flight attendant to wake you before the descent begins.) If you are traveling with an infant or young child, do not allow the child to sleep during descent. Give the child a bottle or a pacifier to suck on—it will help keep the child's eustachian tubes open.

Valsalva Maneuver. If you are unable to unblock your ears by swallowing or yawning, an equalizing technique called the *Valsalva maneuver*, more commonly described as "popping" your ears, can help.

This remedy is an attempt to force air into the back of the nose. To "Valsalva," the American Academy of Otolaryngology recommends that you perform these steps:

1. Pinch your nostrils shut.
2. Take a mouthful of air.
3. Using your cheek and throat muscles, force the air into the back of your nose as if you were trying to blow your thumb and fingers off your nostrils.

When you hear a pop in your ears, you have succeeded in equalizing the pressure inside and outside your ears. It may be necessary to repeat this maneuver several times during the plane's descent. Sometimes you may need to continue this equalizing technique after landing.

Use only the muscles of your cheeks and throat to force the air—these muscles create just the right amount of pressure. Air that is forced from the lungs or diaphragm may result in too high a pressure, so avoid using the muscles of the chest or abdomen.

Also, do not perform this maneuver if you have a cold or sinus infection. You may spread the infection to your ears.

Decongestants. Many air travelers prefer to use an over-the-counter decongestant or nasal spray about an hour before the plane is about to land. These medications help to shrink the tissues around the eustachian tube and encourage the passage to stay open. You still may need to use the Valsalva maneuver, but your ears may be easier to pop.

If you have allergies or sensitive sinuses, take the medication just before takeoff to help avoid discomfort from the buildup of pressure in your ears.

If possible, avoid flying when you have a severe cold or any other acute upper-respiratory condition. If you cannot postpone your trip, take a decongestant before and during the trip to prevent problems. It may help to take one or two drops of ½ percent phenylephrine (*Neo-Synephrine*) (¼ percent for children) or the oral decongestant pseudo-ephedrine (*Sudafed*).

If your ears are still blocked or you have persistent pain after landing, consult an otologist or otolaryngologist as soon as possible.

Scuba Diving

The changes in atmospheric pressure encountered by scuba divers are much greater than those experienced by air travelers. Therefore, the effect on the ears and hearing is potentially more dangerous.

Divers experience the greatest change in pressure from sea level to a depth of 33 feet. For every foot below the water's surface, the pressure increases slightly less than half a pound per square inch. At 33 feet, the volume of air is reduced by half. After a diver successfully reaches this level, the relative changes in pressure aren't as great.

With proper training, some divers are able to reach 33 feet without experiencing any difficulty in equalizing their ear pressure. Others may be especially sensitive to pressure changes and develop such problems as ruptured eardrums and inner-ear damage.

If you have a cold or upper-respiratory infection, wait until it clears up before diving. Learning how to equalize—or clear—your ears is one of the most basic skills required for safe and enjoyable diving. Typically, several tries are necessary to get the knack of clearing your ears underwater. If you are diving and cannot equalize the pressure early in your descent, do not attempt to go any deeper. Your instructor should show you how to successfully use certain equalizing techniques underwater.

Good diving practices can help prevent aerotitis (barotrauma), including descending at a steady pace, making sure your ears have cleared, and not diving when you have a cold or any other condition that inflames your nasal passages.

Swimmer's ear (external otitis) is the second most common disorder in diving. The prevention of swimmer's ear includes such measures as controlling any skin disorders in the ear canal, removing any accumulated earwax, and avoiding polluted water.

To help maintain the protective natural acid balance inside the ear canal, some divers use a simple vinegar-and-water solution. Mix three teaspoons of water with two teaspoons of vinegar. Place several drops in the ear after diving or swimming.

PREVENTING HEARING LOSS FROM OTHER CAUSES

Infection and drugs that are toxic to the ear have been responsible for many cases of hearing loss in the past. Now that immunization against certain diseases and monitoring of potentially dangerous antibiotics are available, it is possible to prevent hearing loss in many children and adults.

Infection

Much of the hearing loss that once occurred in newborns has been significantly reduced as a result of the widespread vaccination of women against the rubella (German measles) virus. If a woman develops rubella during the first three months of pregnancy, she is at very high risk of bearing a deaf child.

Another infection that can cause hearing loss in a newborn is syphilis. If a pregnant woman suspects that she has a venereal infection, she should alert her doctor. If testing determines that syphilis is present, antibiotics will be prescribed.

Infection with the herpes virus also may increase the risk of hearing impairment in the newborn. A pregnant woman who has an active herpes infection should tell her doctor so that precautions are taken to avoid transmitting the virus to the infant just before or during delivery. When there is a danger of passing this infection to a newborn, a cesarean section is usually recommended.

Neonatal jaundice, commonly called Rh (rhesus factor) disease, can produce deafness and other abnormalities in the newborn. This condition occurs when the mother has Rh-negative blood, the father has Rh-positive, and the child may be born with a blood abnormality that causes severe anemia. With the development of a blood test to determine whether there is an Rh incompatibility, a pregnant mother now can be treated beforehand to prevent her child from getting Rh disease.

During childhood, viral and bacterial infections can lead to sensorineural hearing loss. Meningitis is a major cause of acquired hearing loss, which can range from mild to severe. Among the viral infections that occasionally cause hearing loss are mumps, chicken pox, measles, and influenza.

Drugs

Certain drugs are known to cause temporary or permanent hearing loss. They include the salicylates (particularly aspirin), certain antibiotics, and cisplatin, a drug used in the treatment of cancer. (For more information on medications that are toxic to the ear, see chapter 2.)

If you are taking any medications and have noticed that your hearing has changed or that you have a ringing or buzzing sound in your ear, tell your doctor. Your prescription may be changed or modified to prevent the risk of hearing loss.

Antibiotics from the aminoglycoside group (gentamicin, streptomycin, neomycin) are used to treat severe infection. But when they are administered in high doses, they may cause permanent hearing loss. Doctors who prescribe these drugs must closely monitor the level of medication in their patients' bloodstreams.

Chemicals

Studies of workers who are exposed to various chemical agents and their waste products have shown that some of these compounds have the potential to cause hearing loss. It also appears that some organic solvents may cause greater hearing loss when they interact with excessive noise in the workplace.

Among the organic solvents that have been studied in this regard is trichlorethylene, a solvent used as a degreasing agent by dry cleaners and as a chemical agent in the production of paints, waxes, pesticides, adhesives, and lubricants. One study found that the longer workers were exposed to trichlorethylene, the greater their chance of having an abnormal audiogram.

Toluene, a solvent used widely in many industrial applications and in consumer products, also appears to be potentially toxic to the ear. In another study, Brazilian workers who were exposed to toluene and noise had a 53 percent incidence of sensorineural hearing loss, while a comparison group exposed only to noise recorded a 26 percent incidence. A control group with no noise or toluene exposure had an 8 percent rate of hearing loss. The results of this study indicated that exposure to noise increased the risk of hearing loss by 4.6 times, but when noise exposure was combined with toluene exposure, the risk of hearing loss rose 27.5 times.

Carbon monoxide also has been reported to increase the risk of hearing impairment, specifically the effects of cigarette smoking and high noise levels on hearing. (Carbon monoxide is a major by-product of cigarette smoke.) Researchers at Johns Hopkins University exposed laboratory animals to high noise levels and carbon monoxide that equaled the amount inhaled from smoking a single cigarette. They found that lab rats suffered a 20-decibel permanent hearing loss after one exposure to this combination.

Although additional investigation remains to be done, it seems prudent to avoid smoking when constantly exposed to a noisy environment.

Heavy metals, such as arsenic, mercury, tin, lead, and manganese, also have been shown to produce hearing loss in some workers. Researchers are exploring the interaction of these substances with the hearing mechanism but have yet to understand why metals and organic solvents damage hearing. In the meantime, workers who are exposed to these substances should find out what safety precautions they can take to minimize their risk.

Diet

The role of diet in hearing loss remains controversial. Some experts say that food allergies can contribute to hearing impairment, while other disagree.

Some people with Ménière's disease (see chapter 8), a disorder characterized by fluctuating hearing loss, have tried to prevent further attacks by following certain dietary restrictions. Reducing salt intake and eliminating caffeine are the main cornerstones of this attempt at preventive therapy. Some Ménière's patients claim that such dietary changes have been beneficial, but they have yet to be proven scientifically.

Earwax

When earwax accumulates in the ear canal or around the eardrum, it can produce a temporary loss of hearing. Many people who attempt to remove earwax themselves often end up with a greater accumulation—and sometimes an ear infection as well.

The best way to keep your ears free of wax is to leave them alone. Never use a cotton-tipped swab or any other sharp implement to remove earwax. These objects can push the wax up close to the eardrum, resulting in a loss of hearing. Other risks include perforating your eardrum or irritating the skin of your ear canal and setting the stage for infection.

Your ear has a natural self-cleaning mechanism that keeps wax from building up. Daily washing of the outer ears with a clean washcloth usually prevents any problems.

If you occasionally tend to get wax buildup in your ears, try an over-the-counter earwax softener. Follow the directions on the product label. If the softener fails to remove the accumulated wax and your ears still feel blocked, see your doctor or a hearing specialist.

8

Other Auditory Disorders: Dizziness, Vertigo, and Tinnitus

When your sense of hearing is disrupted, it can seriously affect your ability to communicate. But when you hear persistent noise in your ears or suffer constant dizziness, these sensations can throw you, and your life, into confusion and chaos.

Your inner ear contains the body's organ of balance—the vestibular system—as well the cochlea, the organ of hearing. These two systems are interconnected, so when illness or injury strikes the inner ear, one and often both of these complex systems may be affected.

Dizziness is a general term that may mean vertigo, imbalance, or just a feeling of light-headedness. It may point to a disorder of the inner ear, or it may indicate another problem elsewhere in the body. For example, if you have impaired circulation, you may feel dizzy or faint upon suddenly rising out of a chair. That's because the blood flow doesn't travel up to the brain fast enough.

Motion sickness can also cause dizziness. It occurs when the vestibular system gets a series of mixed messages—for example, when you are riding in a car or sailing on a boat. The motion of the car or boat temporarily confuses the system of balance, resulting in dizziness and nausea.

Dizziness is not a disease but rather a symptom of some other problem that may be affecting the inner ear. To find out what causes these problems, it helps to understand the system that maintains our balance and equilibrium.

THE BASICS OF BALANCE

Balance, like so many other body functions, occurs without any conscious awareness on our part, nor do we fully appreciate exactly what it takes to pull off this balancing act.

Your balance system is a highly complex mechanism that relies on information that your brain receives from three major sources: the eyes, the muscles and joints, and the inner ear. Normally, each of these three systems constantly receives information about your surroundings and sends this sensory input to the brain. As long as the messages are clear and the information from one system matches the messages from the others, your body easily maintains its balance. Here's how the three work together:

- *Vision*. Sensory receptors in the retina at the back of your eyes are sensitive to light. When light stimulates these receptors, they send electrical impulses to your brain to let it know where you (and everything else) are. In other words, your vision allows you to see what is around you in relation to your body.
- *Muscles and joints*. The muscles and joints contain sensory receptors called *proprioceptors* that sense the position of your arms and legs. Changes in these tissues cause nerves to fire, sending this information to the brain. They also tell you if you are standing, walking, sitting, or lying down. Simple things, such as the pressure of your foot on a surface—even the stretching of a leg muscle—all get relayed to your brain. The information is received and registered, and you "know" where and in what position your arms and legs are without having to look.
- *Inner ear*. The vestibular (balance) system of your inner ear provides your brain with information about the direction and speed at which your head is turning and about gravity. The system is housed in the bony labyrinth inside your inner ear; sensory receptors in the inner semicircular canals and chambers detect any changes in motion and position. They let the brain know if you are starting or stopping, speeding up or slowing down, are upside down or right side up.

Matching up the Information

If your inner ear's vestibular system is working properly, the nerve impulses from your right ear match those from your left ear when they reach the brain. The information coming from your vision, your joints and muscles, and your vestibular system must convey the same message to the brain. If the information does not match, your brain may become confused and then you feel dizzy.

Of course, a bout of dizziness doesn't necessarily mean that you have an inner-ear disorder. A problem with your vision or your muscles and joints can cause dizziness as well. One cause, related to vision, is wearing a new pair of bifocal lenses for the first time. Adjusting to the different prescription may interfere with your normal vision and leave you feeling dizzy. A similar problem can occur if you rapidly develop cataracts. The change in vision can make you feel off balance.

Motion sickness, too, can make you feel unbalanced. This is a condition in which one part of you senses motion while another part gives conflicting information. For instance, your joints and muscles tell you that your feet are firmly planted on the deck of a boat a mile from shore. But the information sent from your inner ear insists that you are moving. Because this information doesn't match, you may feel dizzy and nauseous.

In Ménière's disease, changes occur in the fluid balance of the inner ear. This can make you feel very dizzy. Infections of the inner ear, such as labyrinthitis and vestibular neuritis, also can quickly alter vestibular function and produce the same effect.

VARIETIES OF DIZZINESS

More than 90 million Americans have experienced dizziness or a balance problem at least once during their lifetimes, according to the National Institute on Deafness and Other Communication Disorders.

When visiting a doctor with a complaint of dizziness, most people express it in vague terms: "I feel dizzy." But such a general statement offers a physician very little information as to the possible cause of your problem.

The word *dizzy* is a descriptive term that many people use when they feel off balance in some way. A cold sufferer with a stuffy head or someone with infected sinuses may complain of feeling dizzy. Another person may feel faint or light-headed when standing in the midst of a hot, crowded room. Someone who enters a dimly lit restaurant may suddenly have a fear of falling, or a feeling of disequilibrium.

Many other conditions or activities can produce dizziness. Engaging in strenuous exercise in hot weather without drinking enough fluids can cause dehydration and a resultant dizziness. Consuming too much alcohol can make anyone feel dizzy and disoriented. A case of influenza, a head injury, and even allergic reactions can produce dizziness. Some people get a sense of confusion and light-headedness as a result of medications they are taking.

If you feel disoriented enough to see a physician, it's important to describe exactly how you feel to the doctor—in other words, explain how the dizziness affects you in detail. The physician needs your description of the experience and any symptoms that accompanied the episode to determine the cause of the problem. The origin of some types of dizziness may be relatively easy to identify, while others may require sophisticated tests to assist the doctor in making a diagnosis.

In general, the symptom of dizziness falls into one of four major categories:

- cardiovascular or circulatory problems
- neurological disorders
- anxiety or depression
- vertigo

Cardiovascular and Circulatory Problems

Suddenly feeling faint, giddy, or light-headed can be a form of dizziness called syncope or near-syncope, a problem that arises from a decreased flow of blood and oxygen to the brain, for whatever reason.

Many of us have occasionally experienced a temporary feeling of dizziness after jumping out of bed in the middle of the night to make a quick trip to the bathroom. Any interference with the circulation of blood as it flows up through the neck to the brain can produce this postural dizziness, including a sudden change in position, hardening of the arteries (arteriosclerosis), an arrhythmia or irregular heartbeat, arthritis in the neck or upper spine, and the use of some medications to lower blood pressure.

A condition that commonly affects older people is *orthostatic hypotension*. In this condition, blood pressure drops quickly after the person rises suddenly from a bed or chair, resulting in faintness or dizziness. It is possible to avoid this by simply taking enough time to change your position. Certain antihypertensive medications, especially the beta-blockers and vasodilators, may play a role in producing orthostatic hypotension.

Fainting also may be brought on by a less common phenomenon that can occur in the nervous system, a *vasovagal attack*. In such an attack, the blood vessels in the legs suddenly lose their muscle tone and cause blood to pool in the legs and trunk, thus reducing the flow of blood to the brain.

To restore normal circulation to the brain and dispel the dizziness, it's recommended that you sit down and place your head between your knees.

Neurological Disorders

Disequilibrium, or imbalance, can also be due to the neurological disorders that affect the parts of the brain concerned with balance—the brain stem, cerebellum, and cerebrum.

The nerves that provide the electrical pathways from the three major balance information sources—the eyes, muscles and joints, and the inner ear—also may stop working properly. The sudden failure of any one of these systems can totally disrupt your stability. Over the long term, it is possible to overcome the loss of one of these systems, but if you were to lose two or all three balance systems (even if the loss is only partial), the multisensory deficit would seriously affect your sense of equilibrium.

A classic example of a person with such a multiple sensory deficit is an elderly person with cataracts, some hearing loss, and decreased sensation in the feet and legs caused by peripheral neuropathy from diabetes or other diseases. The excessive use of alcohol can also complicate the situation. This person's ability to retain balance has probably deteriorated so much that getting up to use the bathroom in a dark house at night may cause a serious bout of dizziness.

By keeping a light on at night, it's possible to provide additional information to the eyes to compensate for losses in other areas.

Anxiety or Depression

Feeling anxious or depressed, or both, may produce a vague sort of light-headedness that some people describe as dizziness. Hyperventilation, or breathing rapidly when you are anxious, can bring on dizziness. This occurs because the rapid shallow breathing causes your lungs to exhale a larger amount of carbon dioxide than normal. When the concentration of carbon dioxide in your blood falls below a certain level, you get tingling in your fingers and toes and may feel lightheaded.

If this happens, you can correct the problem by slowing down your rate of breathing or by the old trick of breathing into a paper bag.

Vertigo

Vertigo is an illusion of motion. You may be standing still and feel that the room is spinning, or you may feel that you are spinning in a stationary room. This disturbed sense of motion is probably due to vertigo, a disorder that usually arises from a disturbance in the vestibular or balance system of the inner ear.

The vestibular system constantly provides the brain with information about your head position, while taking the effect of gravity into account. When the vestibular system stops working properly, it misinterprets or miscodes the position information it receives. As a result, the signals get scrambled and the brain thinks that there is motion when no motion has occurred. A number of conditions can cause this confusion of the balance system, including head injuries, infection, degenerative changes from aging or disease, tumors, excessive use of alcohol, medications, and organic chemicals.

Vertigo often is associated with nausea, vomiting, and an involuntary rapid motion of the eyes called nystagmus. The eye movements of nystagmus reflect an attempt of the brain to correct the problem and realign the vision to normal.

Vertigo also may be linked to problems of the central nervous system or inner ear, and may signal the presence of a serious illness. Multiple sclerosis, stroke, epilepsy, encephalitis, tumors, or an aneurysm can cause vertigo, for example.

Dizziness or Vertigo: Getting a Diagnosis

Because vertigo and dizziness are associated with so many different conditions, it is essential to seek a medical evaluation to learn the cause of your problem.

The first step is to see your family doctor or internist for a complete physical examination. During the first part of the visit, your doctor will ask you to recount any symptoms that occurred when you felt dizzy as well as any events that may have played a role in causing the problem. This aspect of the visit—the history—often holds the key to your diagnosis.

The doctor will also look for clues during the physical examination. In order to rule out any cardiovascular causes, the physician will look for evidence of hypertension or a cardiac arrhythmia, among other things. The workup should include a complete head and neck exam and a neurological evaluation.

Symptoms of Inner-Ear Disorders

VISION

- Objects jump or seem to move (silverware "jumps" off table, stairs "swing").
- Reading is difficult (print moves, vision blurs or doubles, words or letters switch).
- Writing may be difficult.
- Lights glow or emit rays; glare is intensified.
- Tendency to look down. Discomfort increases when you focus at a distance.
- Night blindness increases.
- Depth perception is poor.
- Moving or flickering lights may be disturbing.

HEARING

- Hearing can fluctuate, be lost completely, or be unaffected.
- Distortions such as popping, clicking, or buzzing can occur.
- Noisy environments may be acutely uncomfortable, to the point of making you feel sick.
- The ears may feel full.

NAUSEA

- Continual or intermittent nausea (or occurs only in morning or as fatigue increases)
- A "hangover" feeling or seasick sensation in the head and/or stomach
- Motion sickness

MEMORY

- Poor memory
- You may forget what you are talking about, or grope for words.
- Confusion, disorientation, inability to comprehend directions or instructions

COORDINATION

- Clumsiness (dropping things, difficulty threading needles)
- Sensation of heavy weights on the head
- The center of balance is off.
- Muscle and joint pain
- Balance may be normal (compensation with vision or touch).
- Rocking sensation (as if you're in a rowboat)
- Difficulty walking straight
- Slurred speech

EMOTIONS

- Loss of self-reliance, self-confidence, or self-esteem
- Distraction, anxiety, phobias, or panic attacks
- Depression

OTHER

- Headaches
- Discomfort caused by temperature changes, pressure changes, and wind currents
- Symptoms worsened by high altitude
- Fatigue—everyday tasks are exhausting
- Violent whirling sensations (vertigo), nausea, vomiting

Reprinted courtesy of the Vestibular Disorders Association, Portland, OR.

During the neurological exam, the physician will check the function of your cranial nerves, including vision, hearing, balance, facial motion, as well as mouth and tongue motion. Your gait, stance, and coordination are evaluated, too. The physician will observe your eyes to see if there is any abnormal eye motion (spontaneous nystagmus) and do some position testing to see if that reproduces your symptoms.

The Romberg test also tests basic neurological function. In this test, the physician will ask you to stand up with your feet together, first with your eyes open, and then with your eyes closed. You also may be asked to try some heel-to-toe walking, both with eyes open and closed.

How you respond to these tests helps the physician evaluate whether your problem is in your balance system or elsewhere in the body. If the examination offers no conclusive information, your physician will refer you to a specialist for further tests.

If the specialist suspects that a tumor, vascular abnormality, or central nervous system disease such as multiple sclerosis is causing the vertigo, evoked response audiometry and an MRI (magnetic resonance imaging) scan can aid in making a diagnosis. Computerized tomography (CT) scans also may be used.

Some diseases, such as diabetes, hyperthyroidism, and syphilis, may disrupt the electrolytes in the body and cause some imbalance. Laboratory tests can help determine the presence of these disorders.

Some kinds of dizziness and vertigo are temporary and can be attributed to a specific cause, such as infection or head injury. In other cases, the cause of the dizziness may be difficult to identify.

VESTIBULAR DISORDERS

Vestibular or inner-ear problems can frequently cause severe dizziness or vertigo, affecting people of all ages. These disorders can be frightening, even overwhelming, and can bring on a wide range of symptoms that vary in severity from mild to devastating. Recovering from a vestibular injury may be a slow process. Sometimes the dizziness may disappear and then recur over a period of years.

Benign Positional Vertigo

A young woman skiing down a steep slope fell and struck her head. Getting back up, she continued skiing without any obvious symptoms. Two weeks later, she began feeling dizzy, especially when she moved her head. She also began to have difficulty remembering things, and organizing her workday became more and more difficult. Following a medical evaluation and testing, she was diagnosed as having posttraumatic benign positional vertigo. After several weeks of vestibular rehabilitation therapy, her symptoms gradually abated.

One of the most common causes of vertigo is a condition known as *benign positional vertigo*. Trauma to the head is usually responsible, followed by infection and degeneration of some structures of the inner ear. Hearing loss does not accompany this condition, which usually has a sudden onset.

The sensation of spinning (vertigo) is the major problem—especially when the head is moved to a certain position. Usually, the spinning feeling is precipitated by rolling over to the affected side while in bed. Other positions that may bring on the spinning sensation are sitting or standing up, stooping over, or tilting the head back to look up.

The dizziness occurs when tiny crystals called *otoconia*, which sit on the balance-sensitive organ inside the inner-ear chambers, are injured or destroyed by the trauma. Pieces of the crystals break off and fall down into an area of the semicircular canal—an area where they are not supposed to be. As these crystals float around with certain head motions, they tend to brush against the sensory receptors in the semicircular canal. When this floating debris stimulates the sensors in the canal, it causes a spinning sensation.

Typically, the vertigo occurs about 10 to 20 seconds after the appropriate head motion, lasts about a minute or so, and then disappears. If the motion is repeated again shortly afterward, the vertigo reoccurs, but not as much as the first time. After a period of rest, if the same motion is repeated, the vertigo comes back again in full force.

Benign positional vertigo is a temporary condition that is usually self-limiting. Many people recover after a period of weeks or months, when the crystal particles eventually either fix themselves in place or dissolve. However, in some cases the vertigo may persist and further treatment may be necessary. Among treatment options are medication, vestibular therapy, and sometimes surgery.

Infections of the Inner Ear: Labyrinthitis and Vestibular Neuritis

A middle-aged teacher awakened one day and felt the room spinning around her. When she tried to get up again, the spinning sensation returned, along with nausea. Within seconds, she was in the bathroom, vomiting. After lifting the window shades, she found that she couldn't tolerate bright light. Feeling tired and disoriented, she lay down and felt the vertigo return when she moved her head slightly. When the symptoms didn't clear up in a few days, she called her doctor. The diagnosis: vestibular neuritis, a viral infection that affects the vestibular nerve in the ear. The physician prescribed rest and decongestants. She recovered completely within six weeks.

An inflammation of the inner ear is usually the result of a viral infection that invades part or all of this innermost region of the ear. When both the hearing (cochlea) and balance (vestibular) portions of the inner ear are affected, the condition is called *labyrinthitis*. An infection that settles only in the balance section of the inner ear is known as *vestibular neuritis*.

There also is a form of bacterial labyrinthitis that tends to occur less commonly, but when it strikes, it can be much more severe than the viral form of the infection. Bacterial labyrinthitis can permanently destroy hearing and cause severe vertigo.

The term *labyrinthitis* is often loosely used to describe transient vertigo that occurs as a result of infection. But if the infection doesn't affect the ability to hear in some way, then it isn't labyrinthitis, but vestibular neuritis—or an inflammation of the vestibular nerve.

The symptoms of vestibular neuritis are exactly the same as those of viral labyrinthitis but without the hearing loss. Either form tends to make an acute or sudden appearance. Vertigo may be moderate to severe, with nausea and vomiting. There is usually some nystagmus, an involuntary phenomenon in which the eyes shift abnormally to one side, then move back to their normal position.

In addition to feeling off balance, a person will often experience fatigue and an annoying sensitivity to normal stimuli in the environment, such as light and sound.

Most people who develop an inner-ear infection are disturbed enough by their symptoms to seek medical attention. When the condition is diagnosed, bed rest is recommended until the symptoms begin to disappear.

Rest tends to decrease the symptoms because it reduces stimulation of the vestibular system and brain. By allowing the eyes, muscles and joints, and the balance system of the inner ear to rest, the brain doesn't have to work so hard to adapt and compensate for the missing signals.

Traditionally, people who have acute balance disorders as a result of infection are treated with vestibular-suppressant drugs such as meclizine hydrochloride (*Antivert*) and nausea suppressants like prochlorperazine (*Compazine*) and promethazine (*Phenergan*). However, studies conducted on laboratory models have suggested that vestibular-suppressant drugs also may delay or alter recovery. Animals that were given antiemetics to keep them from vomiting but were encouraged to move around despite their vertigo were found to recover more quickly. Studies are now under way on humans to evaluate these findings.

Depending on the severity of the infection, most cases of viral labyrinthitis and vestibular neuritis resolve completely on their own in a matter of several weeks to several months. Severe cases may take up to six months for recovery.

Toxic Labyrinthitis

Just as certain medications may have an adverse effect on hearing if they are taken in too high a dose, some drugs and even some environmental toxins have the potential to disturb the inner ear's delicate balance system.

Drugs. There are a few preparations within a group of antibiotics known as the aminoglycosides that may affect the vestibular system. Gentamicin, neomycin, and streptomycin are three commonly prescribed medications that may do so.

These medications, usually prescribed for the very ill, must be carefully monitored by the attending physician. Despite precautions to prevent an excessive level of medication from entering the bloodstream, however, some susceptible people may develop a toxic reaction and suffer inner-ear damage.

Anticonvulsants, alcohol, salicylates (aspirin-containing drugs), sedatives, and tranquilizers also may produce some toxicity in the vestibular system.

Workplace toxins. Workers who are exposed to hydrocarbon solvents used in industry may suffer from vertigo and nausea as part of a larger syndrome that affects the entire nervous system.

Swedish researchers reported in 1992 that vestibular symptoms may occur as part of a slowly developing syndrome known as *chronic toxic encephalopathy*. Their studies of workers whose jobs entailed exposure to solvents and petroleum products found that some of the employees developed such symptoms as vertigo, disequilibrium, nausea, and difficulty concentrating.

This syndrome is thought to be somewhat reversible if it is caught during the first few years. However, years of exposure to industrial solvents may lead to such chronic problems as dizziness, memory loss, decreased intellectual acuity, and fatigue.

Among the workers studied were paint mixers, painters, printers, and gasoline truck drivers. The solvents apparently enter the body through the respiratory system and through the mouth and digestive tract.

Allergic Labyrinthitis

A form of allergic labyrinthitis exists, but it is very rare. This disorder may occur in a person with a clearly documented allergy who develops the symptoms of vertigo following exposure to the offending substance.

COMMON ALLERGIES AND VESTIBULAR DISORDERS

Respiratory allergies may increase the symptoms of inner-ear disorders. During allergy season, the offending allergens may cause congestion of the eustachian tube (the drainage tube from the ear) or aggravate some portion of the balance system in susceptible people.

If you develop problems with dizziness in conjunction with allergies, consult your physician. When the symptoms are clearly related to pollens or molds in the environment, then the proper antihistamine will be prescribed to help control the problem. But if your doctor suspects that your vertigo may be due to an inner-ear condition, further evaluation may be necessary.

Ménière's Disease

Ménière's disease, a disorder affecting balance, affects 46 of every 100,000 people. Typically, this condition develops in people age 40 and older. Women have a slightly higher incidence of it than men do.

Ménière's disease was first identified in 1861 by the French physician Prosper Ménière. Up to recently, this mysterious condition has often been overdiagnosed, and general episodes of dizziness were often labeled Ménière's disease. Today, three symptoms are necessary for such a diagnosis: fluctuating hearing loss, recurring vertigo, and noise in the ear (tinnitus).

The underlying cause of Ménière's disease is still not certain, although it is thought that a fluid called endolymph accumulates in the inner ear until the thin sac that holds it ruptures. The buildup of pressure from the excess endolymphatic fluid first irritates the inner ear by increasing the level of tinnitus. The pressure also injures sound-sensing cells in the cochlea and causes a low-toned, nerve-type (sensorineural) hearing loss. When the delicate membranes finally rupture, the fluid spills out and mixes with a different type of fluid, perilymph, which surrounds the inner ear. The result of this intermingling of fluids is immediate vertigo, largely from injury caused to the sensory cells in the inner ear.

It's not unusual for sufferers of Ménière's disease to experience a feeling of fullness in the ear preceding an attack, either by hours or days. Often, the noise of tinnitus also occurs or increases. A fluctuation or drop in the ability to hear is another characteristic sign of an impending attack.

Vertigo—the feeling that the room is spinning—is the main, and most distressing, symptom of Ménière's disease. The sudden, severe episodes of vertigo bring on nausea and vomiting, and may last minutes to hours. Even after the vertigo passes, a feeling of unsteadiness may linger for days.

After an attack, tinnitus and the feeling of pressure in the ear usually disappear, and hearing tends to return to normal. With each succeeding episode, the person's ability to hear is diminished, eventually leading to a severe hearing loss. Rarely, however, does Ménière's disease leave its victim totally deaf.

The course of Ménière's disease is highly unpredictable. A person may have a single attack and never experience another, or may have another bout five years later. Or the disease may become chronic, with daily or monthly attacks occurring over a period of years. Fortunately, most people who suffer from Ménière's disease find that the symptoms resolve on their own over time. Although in most cases the condition occurs only in one ear, about 15 to 20 percent of the time it may develop later in the other ear.

Treatment. No medical cure exists yet for Ménière's disease, but it is possible to control or at least lessen the nausea, vomiting, and vertigo with medication.

Many afflicted people have tried to prevent attacks by turning to a variety of alternative therapies. Heading the list are fluid pills (diuretics) and dietary restrictions, especially reducing salt and eliminating caffeine. Many hearing specialists recommend these particular therapies, based on their clinical observations, but controlled trials have yet to prove them effective.

In the past, it was thought that surgery to halt the vertigo attacks also would stop the progressive hearing loss caused by chronic Ménière's disease. But surgical treatment does nothing to alter this effect of the disease. Surgery can relieve the dizziness that accompanies the disorder, however, and people who have endured many attacks and have tried all of the nonsurgical treatments without any success may choose surgery for relief of their vertigo. Each of the available surgical options is considered relatively safe. Still, every surgical procedure carries some degree of risk.

Three types of surgical treatments are the most commonly performed for Ménière's disease: shunt procedures, vestibular nerve section (neurectomy), and labyrinthectomy.

Shunt procedure. In this operation, an otolaryngological surgeon opens up the drainage sac (endolymphatic sac) to allow the escape of excess fluid from the inner ear. Once the fluid has escaped, normal inner-ear fluid pressure should restore itself, clearing up any dizziness or vertigo.

The success rate for eliminating dizziness during the first year after shunt surgery ranges from 60 to 80 percent. Although originally thought to stabilize and prevent further hearing loss, long-term studies show that the surgery has no effect on the hearing impairment. The shunt procedure is also somewhat controversial. Some investigators claim that this surgery may offer no better results than a similar surgical procedure in which the drainage sac is not exposed or opened.

It is difficult to judge the long-term success of the shunt procedure, because the symptom of dizziness in practically all Ménière's sufferers eventually disappears. The difference is that those who undergo the surgery may have a smoother and easier course to that end.

Labyrinthectomy. In this procedure, the balance portion of the inner ear is surgically destroyed to prevent future episodes of vertigo. The working mechanisms of the labyrinth are also removed or destroyed.

A labyrinthectomy is usually performed for Ménière's victims who have the condition in only one ear and who have no useful hearing in that ear. Vertigo may occur for the first few days after surgery, depending upon how much inner-ear function was present. This may be followed by a few weeks of unsteadiness. Fortunately, the central nervous system soon begins to compensate for the loss of the balance organ on one side, and the symptoms begin to subside.

The other ear's ability to "take over" is dependent on age and general condition. If you are under 40, you can expect to experience a fairly quick compensation for your sense of balance. It will take somewhat longer for people from age 40 to 60, but they usually recover. Anyone 60 and older may have a slight, but permanent, feeling of imbalance that comes when they change position abruptly. Compared to the severe dizzy attacks of Ménière's disease, however, any imbalance is minimal.

The success rate for a labyrinthectomy is about 94 percent. The risks of this procedure include about a one-percent chance of injury to the facial nerve, which could result in paralysis of part of the face. It must be remembered, too, that when a labyrinthectomy is performed, the procedure destroys hearing in the involved ear. For this reason, the operation is done only in people who have no useful hearing in that ear.

Vestibular nerve section (neurectomy). The vestibular nerve in the inner ear that carries signals about balance to the brain is surgically cut in the procedure known as a vestibular nerve section, or neurectomy. This operation is performed in people who have useful hearing still remaining in the affected ear. The rationale is to preserve hearing while at the same time stopping the abnormal impulses that go from the inner ear to the brain. When this surgery is performed by a skilled otolaryngological surgeon, it eliminates the dizziness 90 percent of the time.

Among the risks of the procedure are a 5 to 10 percent chance of hearing loss and about a 2 percent risk of injury to the facial nerve.

The symptoms following a vestibular nerve section are identical to those experienced after a labyrinthectomy: an initial attack of vertigo and some unsteadiness during recovery. As with the labyrinthectomy, people over 60 may have lingering unsteadiness for a period of time, or may even find this problem to be permanent.

Before surgery. When you are considering surgery to alleviate the symptoms of chronic Ménière's disease, choose a skilled otolaryngological surgeon who performs these procedures regularly. Carefully discuss with him or her the benefits and risks of the surgery, and be sure to ask what kind of improvement you can expect, as well as:

- How will the procedure be performed—through the inside of the ear or from behind the ear?

- How many days of hospitalization are required?
- Will the symptoms return after surgery? If so, for how long?
- What is the expected recovery time and how long will it take to get back to normal?

OTHER CAUSES OF DIZZINESS AND VERTIGO

Perilymph Fistulas

A perilymph fistula is an abnormal opening that occurs between the inner ear and the middle ear and allows leakage of inner-ear fluids. (For more information, see chapter 2.)

Alcohol

Many people feel dizzy when they drink too much alcohol. The dizziness can range from a light-headed feeling to a staggering or spinning feeling when the alcohol spreads from the blood into the inner ear and changes how the inner ear responds to motion. Again, the brain receives inaccurate messages, thus causing the sense of imbalance. Once the alcohol has left the inner ear, balance is restored.

Long-term excessive alcohol use can actually damage the inner ear, resulting in a permanent balance problem.

Head Injuries

Head injuries also may cause dizziness. In some cases, the dizziness may not appear for weeks or even months after a direct trauma to the inner ear or a concussion of the brain. Most cases of dizziness from a head injury tend to resolve with time.

Motion Sickness

Motion sickness is often the body's response to movement experienced while riding in a car, boat, or plane. If you have ever suffered from motion sickness, you are well aware of its main symptoms: nausea, vomiting, and dizziness.

At this time there is no one drug that prevents or alleviates the symptoms of motion sickness in everyone. Affected travelers may have to try several preparations before they can obtain relief. Two of the more powerful medications are available by prescription only: Meclizine hydrochloride (*Antivert*) is an antihistamine that suppresses the balance function and thus decreases the effects of motion; scopolamine (*Transderm-Scop*), which also suppresses balance function, is administered through the skin via a patch worn behind the ear. Over-the-counter preparations include dimenhydrinate (*Dramamine*), meclizine hydrochloride (*Bonine*), diphenhydramine (*Benadryl*), and cyclizine (*Marezine*).

Many of these drugs can cause drowsiness. Scopolamine, although more effective than over-the-counter preparations, especially must be used with caution. When scopolamine is taken for longer than three days, it may cause such side effects as blurred vision and dry mouth. Children, people with glaucoma, pregnant women, and elderly travelers with impaired liver or kidney function should avoid scopolamine.

Travel tips. If you prefer not to take any of these preparations, there are practical things you can do to avoid motion sickness.

If on a boat, use the horizon as a point of reference to remind your brain that it is only the surface on which you are standing that is actually moving. Once you "realize" that your leg muscles aren't moving, but that you are really being swayed back and forth, your brain can make sense of the mixed messages it is receiving. By fixing your gaze on the shore, your vision can override—that is, ignore or understand—the messages coming from your muscles and joints. Once you make this adjustment in your brain, your motion sickness will vanish. On longer voyages, this is known as "getting your sea legs." It also helps if you avoid eating heavy meals or drinking alcohol.

In a car, sit up straight and gaze out at distant points on the horizon. Motion sickness on a plane is more difficult to resolve because the aircraft often travels through a cover of clouds. But if the skies are clear, look out the window and stare at the horizon.

One harmless suggestion is to consume two capsules of powdered ginger before traveling. Medical research teams in Britain, the United States, and Denmark conducted separate studies on the effect of ginger on motion sickness and found that the root actually curbed symptoms in some people. The researchers aren't sure how it works, but some researchers believe that ginger may stabilize the stomach, whereas others speculate that it somehow affects the workings of the inner ear.

MAKING A DIAGNOSIS: VESTIBULAR TESTING

An entire battery of tests is available to check the function of the vestibular or balance system. These include electronystagmography, computerized rotation testing, and computerized posturography.

Electronystagmography

The basic screening test used to assess the balance system is electronystagmography (ENG). The responses produced in an ENG test series help to locate the area of the vestibular system that may be causing your vertigo or dizziness.

First, small electrodes are taped to the skin around your eyes. These are attached to equipment that records your eye movement as you gaze at a moving object or shift your vision in certain ways. Eye motion—which is controlled by a system of inner-ear responses (vestibular-ocular reflexes)—indicates how well the inner ear is working. When the vestibular-ocular reflex is disturbed, a distinct eye movement called nystagmus results. Nystagmus is a slow drifting of the eyes away from an object, followed by a quick recovery back to the line of sight. The ENG tests can accurately measure this eye motion.

Further ENG tests include the *tracking test*, in which your eye movements are recorded while you follow a slowly moving object; the *positional test*, which places you in different positions and changes your orientation to the environment; and the *optokinetic test*, which requires you to gaze at a rotating drum while your eye movements are registered.

Another procedure, called *caloric testing*, involves placing warm and then cold water in the ear canal, thus stimulating the inner ear's vestibular system. Changes in temperature may provide enough stimulation to bring about nystagmus.

The specialized equipment used in ENG testing records your eye movements on a graph. By analyzing the pattern and the characteristics of the test results, your physician can determine whether your vertigo originates in the inner ear or is due to a problem in the central nervous system.

Computerized Rotation Testing and Posturography

Two new tests of balance function are *computerized rotation testing* and *computerized posturography*. These tests are so new that researchers have yet to determine exactly how useful they are for routine testing of people with suspected balance disorders.

Computerized rotation testing. In *computerized rotation testing*, you sit on a rotating chair. As the chair moves, the equipment records your eye motion as you look at different objects. Your different responses as you rotate to the right or to the left can provide valuable information on how the inner ear is functioning.

Computerized posturography. *Posturography* (sometimes called moving platform testing) records information about your balance in relation to your movement and the sensory output from the eyes, muscles and joints, and inner ear.

To begin the test, you stand on a platform that is surrounded by a three-sided enclosure. At times, visual patterns or clues are presented on the walls of the enclosure. These motionless or fixed visual patterns move with your body motion. The platform also can tilt or move forward or backward. As you shift your weight in response to the motion or to the visual stimuli, sensors in the platform record and analyze how you are moving. If you close your eyes, or if the visual information being presented on the sides of the enclosure corresponds to the sway of your body, the device records and analyzes this input.

By isolating and analyzing the function of vision, proprioception (muscles and joints), and the vestibular system, computerized posturography may be able to explain why your balance is awry.

Inconclusive Test Results

During the early stages of some vestibular disorders, the history, physical exam, and vestibular test results may be inconclusive in pinpointing the cause or location of your balance problem. When your symptoms persist and there is no clear diagnosis, your doctor may need to reexamine you and have you undergo further testing or reevaluations. In this event, the results of your first evaluation will be used as a baseline for comparison with the later findings. Sometimes, the information obtained from both test reports is helpful in finally making a diagnosis. If your balance problem persists, you may need a second opinion.

THERAPY FOR VESTIBULAR DISORDERS

If you have a vestibular injury or balance disorder, simply turning your head can create distressful symptoms of nausea and dizziness. To prevent further unsettling symptoms, it's natural to avoid as much movement as possible. But scientists are finding that some people who undergo vestibular therapy, a specialized type of physical therapy, often do much better than those who stick to more conventional treatments.

Research in this area is in its early stages, but one study that evaluated the effect of individual custom-designed vestibular exercises showed that 85 percent of the participants had reduced symptoms after therapy. Nine percent reported no change, and 6 percent said their symptoms increased.

Another study compared the effectiveness of vestibular therapy, general conditioning exercises, and antivertigo medication in a group of people with benign positional vertigo disorder. After six weeks of treatment, the severity of dizziness was reduced in all three groups, but balance improved only in those who were given balance training exercises as a part of the rehabilitation program.

Balance Training

Vestibular rehabilitation therapy exercises are tailored to the individual needs of each participant. Before treatment begins, a therapist will assess your posture, balance, and movement and the mechanisms you have developed to adapt to your dizziness problem. The therapist then demonstrates a series of exercises and shows you how to repeat them correctly. Educational materials are supplied to help reinforce what you have learned and to assist you in continuing the exercises at home. The training also emphasizes better ways to move and maintain your balance. You learn how to retrain your control and sense of balance. The exercises are designed to stimulate and enhance the body's normal adaptation to changes in posture, movement, and activity.

Researchers have found the preliminary findings of vestibular therapy to be encouraging. It is hoped that this form of therapy can be applied successfully to most people who suffer from vestibular disorders.

TINNITUS

An agitated 50-year-old man complained to his doctor: "On February 23, around six o'clock in the evening, I began hearing this strange, continuous noise in my head. It hasn't gone away for a month, and it's making my life miserable."

Hissing, ringing, or roaring noises in the ears may bother us occasionally for no apparent reason and then disappear. Unfortunately, this condition, called tinnitus, may persist for a long period of time or even permanently in some people.

Tinnitus may be something that you notice only gradually. Or it may occur so suddenly that the date, time, and circumstances surrounding the beginning of the noise become etched in your memory, as with the patient mentioned above.

Men and women of all ages can be affected by tinnitus, but it is most common among older people. An estimated 50 million American adults suffer from some degree of tinnitus.

Persistent noise in the ears is not a disease, but is a symptom of some other underlying problem with the hearing mechanism. Presbycusis, or age-related hearing loss, is a major cause of tinnitus. A head injury, certain medications, tumors, and even some neurological disorders can produce tinnitus. Sometimes, tinnitus develops for no obvious reason.

Types of Tinnitus

Most people with tinnitus hear a noise in their heads that no one else can hear. Called *subjective* tinnitus, this is the most commonly occurring form. About 97 percent of all the people who complain of noise in their ears have subjective tinnitus.

Another type, known as *objective* tinnitus, is far less common and represents 1 to 3 percent of all tinnitus cases. The objective form is distinguished by the fact that other people can hear the noise as well.

One cause of objective tinnitus is blood flow through the ear or neck region that gives off a pulsating sound as it courses through certain areas of blood vessels. Others include an aneurysm—a swollen, weakened section of a blood vessel—or atherosclerosis—a buildup of debris that narrows the artery wall. Both can produce tinnitus with a char-

Causes of Tinnitus

OUTER EAR
- Earwax
- Foreign object
- External otitis (swimmer's ear)

MIDDLE EAR
- Infection
- Perforated eardrum
- Otosclerosis
- Dislocation of the ossicles
- Tumor
- Arteriovenous malformation
- Aneurysm in the carotid artery

INNER EAR AND THE BRAIN STEM
- Sensorineural hearing loss (from aging, noise, trauma, and all other causes)
- Labyrinthitis
- Ménière's disease
- Perilymphatic fistula
- Acoustic neuroma
- Spontaneous acoustic emissions
- Multiple sclerosis
- Seizures
- Medications
- Head injuries

acteristic sound that matches the heartbeat. When there is a tumor in the ear, blood circulation to the area increases and may produce a rush of sound. This noise—called a *bruit*—can be heard through a stethoscope placed over the ear or upper neck.

Contractions of the tiny muscles of the middle ear or of the palate also may produce a clicking or popping noise that can be heard by others. These rapid, repetitive noises go in bursts of a few seconds.

Spontaneous acoustic emissions—or occasional sounds that a normal ear can produce without any apparent reason—have been picked up and registered by a microphone placed in the ear canal. The sounds that are emitted are rarely heard or perceived by the person or by a listener.

Diagnosing Tinnitus

Most people who develop a persistent ringing or noise in their ears visit their general practitioner first in the hope of finding immediate relief. When the problem continues or worsens, they usually seek the help of an otologist.

The specialist will take a history to determine whether the noise is in one or both ears, how long you've experienced the sound, what it sounds like, when it began, and if you are having difficulty hearing. He or she will ask if you have any other problems, such as dizziness, and what medications you may be taking. A physical examination of the ear, nose, and throat will be performed to look for any physical signs of the disorder. The doctor also may perform a neurological examination. If the noise is pulsatile, the specialist may listen to your neck with a stethoscope. A history of head injuries or loud noise exposure may help determine the cause of the problem.

If the office evaluation fails to pinpoint the source of the tinnitus, the specialist will order hearing tests. Very often, the results of the audiogram show a hearing loss in both ears that is associated with tinnitus.

When there is tinnitus in only one ear, or if the hearing test is normal, further diagnostic tests may be necessary. Auditory brain-stem response testing, magnetic resonance imaging (MRI), and computerized tomography (CT) may be required. These special tests are conducted to rule out more serious causes of tinnitus, such as an acoustic neuroma, multiple sclerosis, or neurological or circulatory disorders.

If testing reveals a treatable problem, such as otosclerosis (a bone disorder that affects the middle ear), your doctor will explain the treatment options that are available (see chapter 2).

Treating Tinnitus

Unfortunately, in many instances there is no cure for tinnitus. Sometimes the noise disappears on its own, but usually it fades into the background and becomes noticeable only under periods of stress, fatigue, or intense quiet. It tends to be more of an annoyance than a major problem for most people.

Over-the-counter medications or prescription drugs can also produce tinnitus. You may be surprised to find that aspirin or a nonsteroidal anti-inflammatory agent is responsible for the problem. Certain antibiotics and quinine derivatives also may cause tinnitus. If a medication is thought to be causing the problem, your doctor will ask you to eliminate the drug and substitute another, if possible.

Sometimes a medically or surgically correctable problem is found, and proper treatment relieves the tinnitus.

Drugs. Currently, there are no drugs that are approved by the FDA for the treatment of tinnitus. Many have been studied but have not been shown to be beneficial, including lidocaine, which produced only temporary relief and had serious side effects such as slurred speech, amnesia, and fainting. Anticonvulsant medications also have been investigated but were found to be only slightly effective in reducing tinnitus.

The antianxiety drug alprazolam (*Xanax*) has been prescribed by some doctors for patients with tinnitus, and some people have reported that the medication has been helpful. However, alprazolam carries the risk of psychological dependency when it is used for a long period of time.

Electrical nerve stimulation. Electrical nerve stimulation, a still-experimental technique, sends a small charge of electricity into the inner ear and auditory nerve in the hope that it will override the defect causing the tinnitus.

In a few isolated cases, electrical nerve stimulation has helped relieve tinnitus. But the majority of people who have tried this form of therapy have experienced no relief; others have reported that their tinnitus worsened after the stimulation.

Tinnitus maskers. A tinnitus-masking device contains an amplifier that emits a steady band of white noise, which substitutes for the noise of the tinnitus. As an added feature, many tinnitus maskers are combined with a hearing aid. Some people prefer the masking sound because it effectively drowns out the disturbing noise coming from their own ears. Also, unlike the persistent drone of tinnitus, it's possible to adjust the volume of the masker sound.

A tinnitus masker requires a visit to an audiologist. The audiologist will ask you to listen to a series of tones until a tone is located that matches the frequency level of your tinnitus. You are then custom-measured for a unit that looks somewhat like a hearing aid and is worn the same way.

Buy only tinnitus-masking devices that are approved by the FDA: A masker that is too loud or overstimulates the ear has the potential to cause hearing loss. To date, long-term use of an FDA-approved masker has not been found to be damaging.

Not every tinnitus sufferer benefits from a masking device. One problem is that exactly matching the masking sound to the tinnitus noise level is tricky. If you are having a stressful day, your tinnitus may sound louder to you, in which case the masker would not be as effective. And the frequency and intensity of tinnitus noise can change from day to day.

Some tinnitus maskers are touted as producing a posttinnitus masking effect—that is, a disappearance of the tinnitus after removal of the masking noise. This period of freedom from interior noise is short-lived, however. For reasons that are not understood, the noise may go away briefly—for a few seconds, minutes, or occasionally for a few hours—only to return later.

Small electrical devices called bedside maskers also are available. These units produce a distracting form of background noise. Some use tapes of soothing environmental sounds, such as rainfall or the ocean's muted roar, to create a different sound ambience. Some tinnitus sufferers prefer to fall asleep to these sounds, while others may just leave a radio on at night. Selecting an FM station that plays soft music or even setting the dial between two stations to pick up soft static often helps reduce the annoying awareness of tinnitus at night.

Diets. Multiple dietary therapies have been claimed over the years to relieve tinnitus. To date, none of these regimens has been proven effective. Certain dietary restrictions may help some people, though, and warrant a trial period. Elimination of caffeine, alcohol, and nicotine is the basic focus of these restrictions, because these substances may worsen tinnitus.

Relaxation and noise avoidance. As mentioned previously, tinnitus has a tendency to fluctuate with changes in a person's level of fatigue, stress, and exposure to outside noise. When these changes occur, it doesn't necessarily mean that the tinnitus is getting worse. The noise usually settles back to its original baseline once the disruption has been resolved.

Obviously, reducing stress and anxiety are the most effective measures you can take to decrease the intensity of your tinnitus. Being around excessively loud noise or even staying in a very quiet area also may exacerbate tinnitus, so it is best to avoid these extreme situations.

To find some relief from stress, you may decide to try the following:

- relaxation techniques
- biofeedback
- yoga
- regular exercise
- adequate rest
- hypnosis

Most people eventually cope with their tinnitus and learn to live in peaceful coexistence with it. However, in about one percent of all tinnitus sufferers, the problem becomes disabling. For these people, psychological counseling may be necessary.

9

Coping with Deafness

Instead of enjoying the happy retirement they had long anticipated, Linda and Fred were on the verge of divorce. The problem was chiefly Fred's inability to handle his hearing loss. At the urging of his family, Fred finally had consented to wear a hearing aid. But the self-consciousness he felt while wearing it, along with a growing feeling of inadequacy over not being able to communicate as before with his wife and friends, eventually led to a crumbling of his self-confidence. Instead of attempting conversations with others, or even viewing a television program on his own, he asked his wife to repeat everything that was said. After a few years of this dependency, her resentment and frustration grew to the point where she considered divorce the only solution. Fortunately, this couple discovered a course on coping strategies for the hard-of-hearing and for the people who live with them. The teacher taught Fred how he could be away from his wife and communicate on his own. He soon saw that he could participate in a conversation, and his self-esteem soared.

Coping with hearing loss isn't simply a matter of buying a hearing aid or assistive listening device and waiting for life to get back to normal. It takes time and effort to learn to use a hearing aid successfully, and people often need to develop other strategies to supplement their understanding of speech. Beyond these technical solutions lie issues that are the hardest to deal with: coming to terms with the emotional suffering and psychological pain of deafness.

LEARNING TO LIVE WITH HEARING LOSS

Whether you are an adult who is experiencing a loss of hearing, or a parent trying to attend to a newly diagnosed hearing-impaired or deaf child, living with hearing loss is a painful process. It means accepting the sense of loss and coping with the inevitable grief that follows.

Adults with Hearing Loss

Marvin, a retired accountant and widower, became withdrawn and depressed. He declined invitations to family gatherings, much to his daughter's dismay. If he did attend social functions, his conversation occasionally seemed inappropriate and disjointed. Eventually, he spoke very little and his interest in his surroundings decreased markedly. His behavior led his daughter to wonder whether her father had developed Alzheimer's disease or some other degenerative disorder. At the urging of his family, Marvin went to his doctor, who quickly discovered that Marvin was healthy physically but was hard-of-hearing. After examination and testing by an audiologist, Marvin was fitted for a hearing aid and shown how to use it. Once he became accustomed to relying on hearing devices, Marvin gradually resumed socializing and enjoying his life.

Adults who develop a loss of hearing often have difficulty in acknowledging that they have a problem. Pride often stands in the way, and years of increasing frustration may go by until help is sought. Marvin, for example, told the specialist who treated him that he was afraid people who knew about his deafness would treat him like "an old man."

Adults who try to conceal a hearing problem may, like Marvin, attempt to bluff their way through conversations, become increasingly withdrawn and depressed, or feign indifference when friends or family try to interest them in excursions, trips, or other social activities. They may increase the volume on the TV or radio to an unbearably loud level, or have trouble speaking on the telephone. They often complain of people "mumbling" and urge family members to "speak up."

These people are really bewildered and frightened by what is happening to them. Sometimes it takes a shock before they realize their plight—the inability to hear the dialogue in a play or film, for example, or the embarrassment that occurs when they misunderstand a conversation or make a gaffe at an important meeting or social gathering.

Once they realize and admit to themselves that they have a hearing problem, they are well on their way to dealing successfully with their impairment.

The coping strategies offered in courses given by community groups and health centers (see appendix C) focus on stress management techniques and the resolving of any problems that arise because of the hearing loss. The major focus is on improving communication skills.

Relearning Basic Communication Skills

People with normal hearing often don't know how to talk to someone with a hearing loss. They typically talk louder, or even shout, which just makes the situation worse. An overly loud voice may annoy the listener, and yelling tends to exaggerate facial expression and distorts what is being said.

On the other hand, all too often hard-of-hearing people don't volunteer the fact that they have a hearing problem. This is a mistake. Most people appreciate being told and will adjust the speed and clarity of their words to help someone converse more easily.

A conversation between a hard-of-hearing person and someone with normal hearing calls for different ground rules. Effective two-way communication can take place when some simple techniques are followed. The participant with a hearing loss needs to use certain listening skills, and the hearing person must adopt specific speaking skills.

Some strategies for improving communication between the hard-of-hearing and those with normal hearing are:

- As stated previously, if you are hearing-impaired, tell others that you have hearing loss. When you admit that you have a hearing problem, neither you nor anyone else will have to pretend the problem doesn't exist.
- Indicate to others how you can best hear them. This may mean asking the speaker to direct his or her voice to your better ear or moving to a quieter part of the room.
- Choose your conversational spot in advance. Sit or stand in a place where the light is behind you so that you can better see the speaker's face. Avoid noisy backgrounds. Position yourself close enough to the speaker so that you can listen and speechread as well.
- Anticipate potential problem situations and plan ways to alleviate any difficulties. If you will be attending a meeting, conference,

lecture, or other event, request an agenda or other related information in advance. Or if you are invited to a party where there will be a number of guests whom you don't know, ask for a short advance briefing. By memorizing people's names and other particulars before the event, you will feel more confident during introductions and in later discussions.

- If you plan to dine at a restaurant, ask for a quiet table on the side or in the corner. Make sure the table is well away from the kitchen, cashier, and bar, because these areas are noisier.
- When actually engaged in a conversation, concentrate only on the speaker and don't allow anything in the background to distract you.
- Be aware of any facial expressions, gestures, or body language that may provide important visual clues to the conversation.
- Don't always interrupt immediately if you don't understand something. Very often, the speaker will repeat the word you missed and you can keep on listening. But if you find that you have missed a significant part of a sentence, ask for a repetition. You can repeat or rephrase what you think you heard and then ask the speaker if that is correct.
- If you aren't keeping up with the conversation, let the speaker know. Don't expect that a puzzled look on your face will alert the speaker that you are off the track. Explain what you thought was said. Then follow up by asking, "Is that right?"
- Don't imply that you've understood a conversation when you haven't. Bluffing is a major cause of problems for people who are hard-of-hearing. You'll feel more confident when you know you have truly understood the communication that is taking place in each conversation, and others will appreciate your honesty. Don't be afraid to ask questions to get all the information you need.
- If you feel too tired to undertake a lengthy conversation, ask if you can talk to the person later. Good listening calls for focused concentration, which can be extremely tiring when done for long periods of time.

If you have normal hearing and are talking to people who are hard-of-hearing:

- Face the hard-of-hearing person directly. Don't turn to the side or talk from another room or when the person's back is turned to you.

- Don't chew gum or eat while talking. Pipes, cigars, and cigarettes are also obstacles to clear understanding. Keep your hands away from your face when talking.
- Ask the hard-of-hearing person what you can do to foster better communication. This may mean moving to a quieter area or to a spot where the light falls on your face and allows the listener to observe your mouth as you talk.
- The noise of a radio, television, air conditioner, or fan can interfere with clear understanding. If you can't turn these appliances off, move to a quieter spot in the room.
- As stated previously, don't shout when talking. Shouting only distorts the speaker's face and makes it nearly impossible for a hard-of-hearing person to understand what is being said. And, if the listener is wearing a hearing aid, a loud voice may be amplified to the point of pain.
- Speak clearly. Slow your speaking pace to moderate. Pause occasionally so that your words are easier to follow.
- If you have been asked to repeat something, and the hard-of-hearing person still doesn't understand, rephrase the sentence. If rephrasing fails to help, write down the essential information.
- Don't change subjects abruptly. Let the listener know you're on another topic.
- Use gestures and facial expression to enhance your speech, but not excessively. Smiling, frowning, shaking your head, and moving your hands can provide effective visual clues.
- Don't talk to others about a hard-of-hearing person who is standing or sitting with you, and never talk around a hard-of-hearing person as if he or she weren't there.
- Be patient and relaxed. By offering encouragement and a positive attitude, you help your listener to feel less frustrated and thus able to follow the conversation with greater ease.

LISTENING AND SPEAKING TECHNIQUES

Speechreading

In the past, observing a person's lip movements in order to better understand what was being said was called *lipreading*. But speech and language experts found that the term was too limiting. Instead of observing only the shape of words coming from a person's mouth, a hard-of-hearing person also looks for facial cues, body language, and conversational clues. Because visual expressions always accompany human speech, the technique of "reading lips" is now known as *speechreading*, which incorporates all the various means of comprehending what is being said.

Speechreading for the partially or completely deaf person requires total concentration on their part. Some master the technique quickly, while others must be highly motivated and willing to practice and persist—sometimes for years. Because observing visual clues to speech is a natural process, many who have a slowly progressing hearing loss begin to speechread without even being aware they are doing it.

Speechreading strategies. Speechreading is not an absolutely surefire way of comprehending every word of a conversation. It's more like filling in the blanks in a difficult crossword puzzle. Even the most accomplished speechreader won't pick up 100 percent of a conversation by visual observation alone. In fact, only about 30 percent of speech information is obtained from lip movements. The rest comes from motion of the mouth and jaw.

Another factor is that some sounds, called homophonous sounds, look identical when pronounced. These sounds include the spoken letters *p*, *b*, and *m*, which look the same on the lips and mouth. Look in a mirror and try saying *pan*, *ban*, *man*—taking care to observe how your lips appear when enunciating each of these words. Someone who is speechreading would have to decide which word is being used, based almost solely on the direction and subject of the conversation.

Invisible sounds are also produced orally with virtually no jaw, mouth, or lip movement. These unseen sounds include *n*, *d*, *t*, *g*, *k*, and *ng*. When a sentence contains a string of these sounds, it can be difficult indeed to get the gist of what is being said.

But certain strategies can be employed to enhance the speechreading technique. In fact, many of the strategies for better listening presented earlier also apply to speechreading. These include positioning yourself so that you can see as well as hear the speaker, and also listening for key words in the conversation.

Some speakers present special listening problems. They speak too quickly, or they may mumble or have very little natural movement of their mouth when they speak. You can ask the fast talker to slow down, but mumblers may not be able to change their manner of speaking. A person with a foreign accent or a speech impediment also is more difficult to speechread.

Following the conversation among a group of people can be especially frustrating. It's best to follow the conversation visually and watch each speaker's face. This way, you can pick up key words as you try to keep up with the group.

Remember that the inflection and flow of a person's voice provide important clues. When a question is asked, the voice tends to rise. A voice becomes somewhat louder, and words are emphasized when an important point is being made. Usually, a natural pause occurs at the point when a speaker is concluding a thought or a story.

Speechreading classes. Speechreading can be self-taught, but some hearing-impaired people may not have enough motivation to develop all the skills they need on their own. For many, the lack of a partner to practice with is sufficient reason for them to seek out a speechreading course.

Classes are available in many communities. To find out where they are offered, contact the audiology or speech pathology department of your local hospital. If you live near a university or college, call the school and ask for the speech and hearing science department. A list of where you can get speechreading lessons nationwide is available from the Alexander Graham Bell Association (see appendix C).

Classes may contain as few as three people or as many as 10. Group classes cost less than individual sessions and may be more effective because participants get a chance to meet other people with similar problems—and can share their own frustrations and solutions. Group members also offer support and encouragement. There are opportunities to practice speechreading in quiet settings with just one other person and in more challenging, noisier situations as well.

Auditory Training

An auditory training program is usually offered with the goal of achieving better listening with the help of a hearing aid. It's a process in which the hearing-impaired person learns to take advantage of all the acoustical cues that are available to the ear. Essentially, it is instruction in how to use any residual or remaining hearing in the most effective way.

Auditory training was originally used in schools for the deaf to make students aware of sounds around them, such as automobiles, running water, doorbells, and barking dogs. But after World War II, auditory training techniques were widely applied in hearing rehabilitation centers for returning veterans.

In this postwar period, some of the first wearable hearing aids were just coming into use. As hearing-impaired servicemen were fitted with the aids, hearing professionals realized that individual training in the proper adjustment of the hearing aid and lessons in *interpreting* what was heard through the device were necessary. In response to this need, an auditory training program was developed that now serves as the model for hearing-impaired people of all ages.

The results of speech discrimination tests—that is, the ability to understand the spoken word—are used to determine the level of auditory training needed. The focus of the auditory training program is on learning to distinguish specific sounds used in speech.

If you are only partially hearing-impaired and understand speech fairly well, very little training may be necessary for you to get the most from your own hearing with the help of a hearing aid. But if you have a low score in speech discrimination and constantly miss words with consonant sounds like *s*, *f*, *p*, *t*, *k*, *h*, *th*, *sh*, *ch*, and *wh*, then your auditory training program would be designed to help you better distinguish words using these sounds.

An audiologist or speech pathologist can work with you to improve your recognition of words that have a similar distribution of vowels and consonants. If you are an adult with a significant sensorineural hearing loss, auditory training won't bring your hearing back to normal, but it can help you to communicate better.

DEAF AND HEARING-IMPAIRED CHILDREN

The parents of a child who has been diagnosed with a significant hearing impairment often feel a deep sense of grief. The initial shock of discovery may also engender feelings of anxiety, inadequacy, guilt, and confusion.

If you are grieving for a child affected in this way, know that this is a normal reaction. As with death, it is necessary to go through a period of mourning while you come to terms with the situation. You will have to discover what the hearing loss means to your child and to your own life and that of your family.

The Importance of Early Diagnosis

▬

One in every 1,000 babies born in the United States is deaf at birth or suffers a severe hearing disorder. According to a panel of experts assembled by the National Institutes of Health in 1993, fewer than half of these children are recognized as being hearing-impaired until their condition has already compromised speech and language development.

The average age for identifying deaf or severely hearing-impaired children in this country is almost three years old, and lesser degrees of hearing loss go undetected even longer. Since the first three years of life are the crucial period for developing speech and language skills, poor hearing at this stage can interfere with communication skills for the rest of a person's life.

The panel recommended the following hearing tests for infants:

- *Otacoustic emissions*. Quick, noninvasive, and inexpensive, this test is done before an infant leaves the hospital.
- *Auditory brain-stem response audiometry*. This test should be done when an infant fails the otacoustic emissions testing. It is technically more difficult, costs more, and takes more time, but has been recommended for screening high-risk infants for more than 15 years.

The sadness you feel may last a long time. But, despite your sorrow, you need to consider the well-being of your child and what he or she must do to eventually develop normal language skills. A hearing-impaired child needs remedial therapy as soon as it's feasible.

Helping the Hearing-Impaired Child

As soon as possible after the diagnosis of a hearing problem in your child, seek out a qualified team of professionals who can determine what needs to be done to help your child develop speech and language skills. The team members may include an audiologist, an otolaryngologist, a speech and language pathologist, a pediatrician, possibly a psychologist experienced in working with the hearing-impaired, and if necessary, an occupational or physical therapist.

Is Your Child Deaf or Hard-of-Hearing?

The term *deaf* usually describes a person with no hearing ability, but most people who are technically deaf have varying, if small, amounts of residual hearing. According to the experts, there are 15 times more hearing-impaired children than completely deaf children.

The federal Individuals with Disabilities Education Act (IDEA) of 1975 distinguishes between *deaf* and *hard-of-hearing* in the following way:

- *Deaf* is applied to a hearing impairment so severe that the child is impaired in processing linguistic information through ordinary or amplified hearing, which adversely affects educational performance.
- *Hard-of-hearing* is applied to a permanent or fluctuating hearing impairment that adversely affects a child's educational performance but that is not included under the definition of *deaf*.

The main distinction centers on the amount of residual hearing that remains and how the child communicates with others. A deaf child may be able to use whatever small amount of auditory function is available, but only as a supplementary way of getting information. For this child, visual skills and strategies—such as speechreading and using sign language—may be the primary way of receiving information from other people.

Several factors play a role in the development of a child who is deaf or hard-of-hearing. Among these are the age of the child when the hearing loss occurred, the degree and type of hearing loss, the cause of deafness, the child's age when training or school programs were begun, the age when the child was fitted with a hearing aid, how well the child does with the hearing aid, and the family environment. The child's style of learning and way of communicating also influence development and the ability to function in social and educational settings.

Because hard-of-hearing children can effectively use auditory information and strategies, they rely primarily on spoken information in communicating with others. Usually this is done with the help of a hearing aid or assistive listening devices.

The audiograms of some children indicate a hearing loss that is so severe it defines them as deaf. Nevertheless, they may be able to function as hard-of-hearing youngsters. Similarly, other children who are technically hard-of-hearing may find that they prefer to be members of the deaf community.

Each hearing-impaired child must be assessed individually, so a special plan should be created to meet your child's needs. His or her capabilities, degree of hearing loss, and ability to function with a hearing aid must all be taken into consideration.

Early-intervention centers can offer guidance and support as you try to maximize your child's potential while at the same time striving to give him or her a normal upbringing. You will be successful the more you are able to put the child's hearing problem into perspective and consider it as just a part of daily living.

What Not to Do. It's easy for well-meaning parents to fall into certain traps in raising a hearing-impaired child. One such pitfall is the danger of overemphasizing the child's educational needs and overlooking equally strong needs to develop socially. A youngster who is not able to relate to his or her peers isn't likely to become a well-rounded, happy adult.

Other parents throw themselves into the management of their deaf child's life and education to the detriment of their family and their own social and emotional needs. Not only does this weaken the strength of the family, which is so crucial to the hearing-impaired child, it also affects the child's siblings and may create resentment that can last a lifetime.

Another potential problem occurs when parents focus so much on the child's use of words and language that every encounter turns into a lesson. Parents have to remember that childhood is also a time to be enjoyed—by both parent and child.

A few parents may reject their hearing-impaired child; many others take the opposite route and are overly protective and caring, to the point where the child feels smothered and helpless. Obviously, neither of these approaches is helpful in the child's overall development.

Teaching the Deaf and Hearing-Impaired Child

A baby with normal hearing will hear language for a year before saying the first word. By the age of 5, the child has a vocabulary of 5,000 to 26,000 words. A deaf child of the same age, however, will have a vocabulary of only 200 spoken or signed words.

As the hearing child proceeds through each grade in school, the lessons help to formalize the language system through reading and writing. However, the average deaf child who relies largely on American Sign Language (ASL) lags far behind in reading and writing skills. This is because ASL has no written form.

It is obvious from these few statistics that the hearing-impaired child needs early exposure to learning language and communication skills. However, just as parents can't rush children with normal hearing into early speech, deaf children also cannot be forced to learn language at an accelerated pace. Their comprehension of language must go through the same learning curve as a normal-hearing infant.

Two main educational approaches are available to the deaf child. One approach, which consists of multiple methods of learning, is called *total communication*. This program includes auditory training, sign language and gesture, as well as the benefits of a hearing aid. With this method, parents especially are encouraged to use all means of communication with their deaf children.

A second educational approach involves teaching the child sign language, which provides the child with a visual language instead of the usual auditory language system. If this type of training is selected, parents (and relatives and friends) need to learn the language in order to communicate effectively with their children.

This is a controversial topic within the deaf community. What is important to remember is that no two children are alike. The choice of which educational program to pursue must be made on an individual basis, taking into account the needs of the child, the family situation, and the availability of resources within the community.

The hard-of-hearing child. Children who have a mild to moderate hearing loss are not necessarily put into preschool programs for the hearing-impaired. Typically, it is recommended that their parents enroll them in a special-needs preschool that concentrates on acquiring language skills. Additional lessons from a speech-language professional may also be needed.

If the child's hearing loss is identified early enough, and the child is fitted with an amplification device, usually the youngster can be placed in classes with normal-hearing children at the beginning of elementary school.

Before enrolling a child in a preschool program, talk to the staff and to the parents of other hearing-impaired children who are already in the program. Ask them about the progress their children are making in both early language use and in socializing with other children. Make certain that the program is designed for hard-of-hearing children (not only deaf children), because there is a difference.

The deaf child. When a child has a severe to profound hearing loss, then a program that fully involves the parents—right from the time of diagnosis—is the recommended approach. Any delay in beginning training can cause a loss of valuable time and put the child even further behind in acquiring basic language skills.

As soon as hearing loss is identified, the deaf child will be given auditory training—instruction in using residual hearing and sound recognition—and then be fitted with a hearing aid. When there is virtually no auditory function, learning other ways to communicate, including sign language, may be necessary. Within three to five years after the child has begun wearing the hearing aid and receiving language instruction, speech and hearing professionals can determine what kind of extra help is necessary. They will consider the child's language development as well as how the child is integrating socially with the family and with youngsters in the same age group.

Children who do well with a hearing aid often can be expected to hold their own in a regular classroom—often with supplementary tutoring and extra help. One form of assistance for more severely hearing-impaired students is the presence of oral interpreters who silently mouth the words said in the classroom, or interpreters who use sign language to repeat the lessons. Another form of help is note taking—a student with normal hearing takes notes on pressure-treated paper and gives the copy to the hearing-impaired student. This allows the hearing-impaired student to fully concentrate on what the teacher or other students are saying, without the extra burden of taking notes.

If a deaf child is not doing well in a regular classroom among normal-hearing children, the parents must investigate other educational options for the child. However, it's impossible to predict in advance what academic difficulties any child may encounter.

AUDITORY TRAINING FOR CHILDREN

Young children who require a hearing aid need special training in how to use the appliance effectively. They may be confused by the many sounds they hear when an aid is first fitted to their ear. Because these sounds may seem to be unwanted noise to them, they must be taught to listen and recognize the sounds that convey important information. Without this instruction, the child could reject the hearing aid and lose the opportunity to develop adequate language and speech skills.

Before a child is fitted for an aid, the auditory training instructor teaches the child what the amplified sounds mean. The instructor relates the sounds to animals, people, places, and objects in the environment. As the child picks up on these sounds, he or she learns to differentiate among them and to identify and make sense of particular ones. Only after this initial training is the child fitted with a hearing aid.

Once the youngster becomes accustomed to the hearing aid, the instructor begins helping the child to recognize words and the sounds that make up speech. Ideally, the child should associate each word with the object it stands for. But many words sound so similar—like *ball* and *bell*—that the teacher may have to work on the separate sounds that make up different words. The child first learns to imitate the words and then to use them in speech.

The rhythm, pitch, loudness, and phrasing of spoken language are also an integral part of auditory training. In order to gain meaning from conversation, the child must recognize the differences in sound cues. For example, a rising inflection at the end of a sentence indicates a question, while a downward inflection indicates that a sentence will terminate. Speechreading is also taught as a regular part of the training curriculum.

The child learns acoustic cues by playing various sound recognition games. Parents are encouraged to take part in these learning activities at home in order to reinforce the training program and carry it over into the child's daily routine.

Educational Options for the Deaf Child

Finding and selecting the best learning environment for a hearing-impaired or deaf child is difficult for any parent. Many considerations are involved, but the most important one is the understanding of the individual child's needs. Next is awareness of the educational services available, and knowledge of how trained professionals can help meet those needs.

Children with mild to moderate hearing loss (and even some with a more severe impairment) may be able to function in a regular classroom equipped with appropriate amplification or assistive listening devices. Youngsters with profound hearing loss may have to attend special schools for the deaf, where they can get specialized speech and language classes.

Understandably, many parents want their child to attend a nearby school with normal-hearing children. However, this may be the worst educational setting for a hearing-impaired or deaf child.

LEARNING TO COMMUNICATE: WHICH SYSTEM IS BEST?

Different schools of thought exist on the philosophy of how hearing-impaired children should learn speech and language communication skills. Each system has its advocates, opponents, and even its extremists. Some members of the deaf community, for example, consider deafness simply a cultural difference and believe that the deaf person should use sign language exclusively.

The deaf can communicate in two basic ways: by oral communication or by manual communication. Another method, total communication, combines both approaches.

Oral Communication

Children who are enrolled in an oral communication program use a hearing aid and receive auditory training. The oral approach relies on the use of the child's residual hearing as the primary basis of exchanging information.

A child's ability to speak is influenced, of course, by the degree of hearing loss and the age at which it occurred. A child who had normal speech and hearing and lost both as a result of illness is a candidate for another kind of oral training, *speech conservation*.

Learning speech conservation helps children (and adults) to be aware of and to correct problems in voice quality that may accompany hearing impairment. A flat tone, or a lack of intonation, for example, often

Educational Rights of the Hearing-Impaired

Since 1975, the law states that every child with impaired hearing has the right to a free, appropriate public education that meets his or her particular needs. This may mean attending regular classes with the necessary support services, obtaining speech therapy, joining auditory training groups, or enrolling in a public or private school for the deaf.

In October 1992, the Department of Education issued policy guidelines clarifying this law for state and local education agencies. The purpose is to ensure that the needs of deaf students are properly identified and met, and that parents are kept informed about any decisions made by public agencies in placing their child in one classroom setting or another.

Under the new guidelines, the school must write an individual education plan that addresses the needs of each individual deaf child.

A child's language, communication, social, and psychological needs all enter into the plan, which includes:

- communication needs and the preferred mode of communication
- linguistic needs
- severity of the hearing loss, and the potential for using residual hearing
- the child's academic level and style of learning
- social needs
- placement preference
- emotional needs
- individual motivation
- cultural needs
- family support

When parents disagree with the school system over a placement decision, they have the right to a due process hearing before an independent hearing officer. Parents who initiate a formal complaint are advised to hire an attorney or an advocate for help with their case.

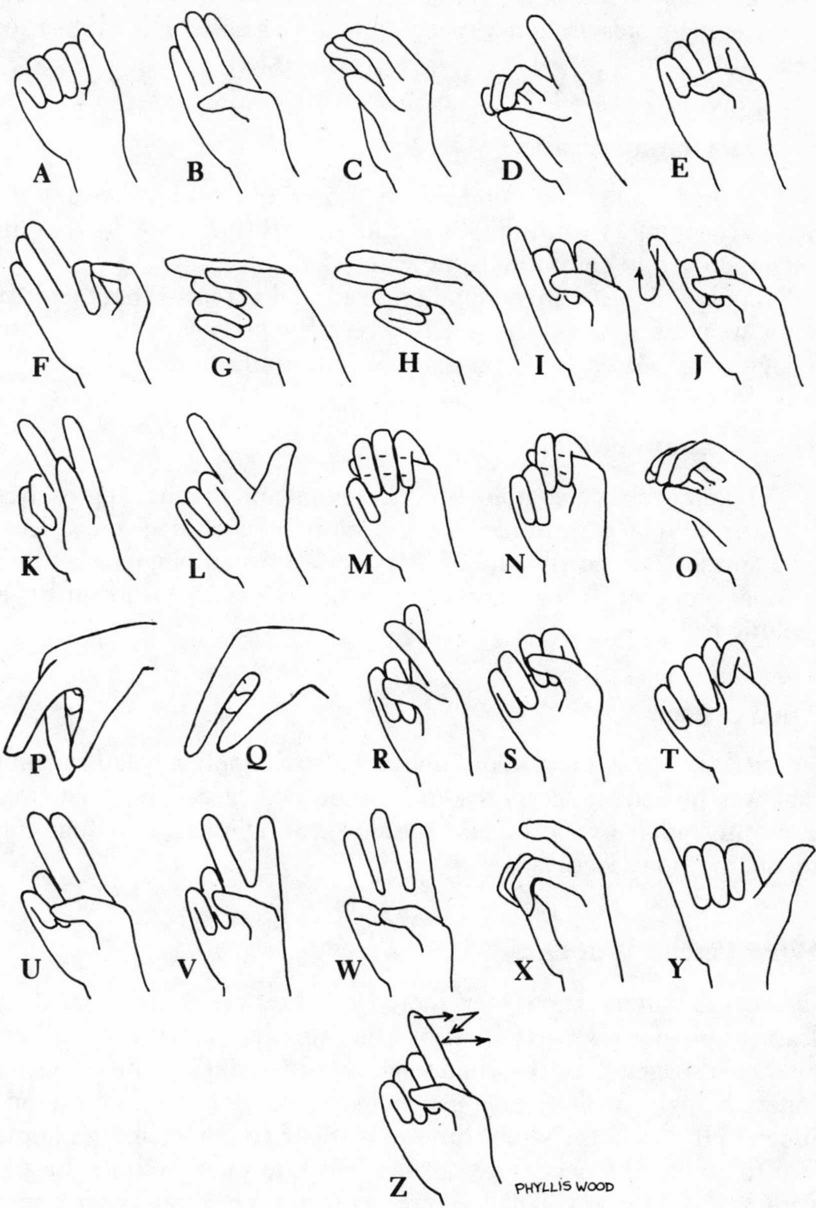

The American manual alphabet

gives a deaf person's speech a monotonous sound. Talking too loudly and slurring words are other speech problems associated with hearing loss.

Manual Communication

A manual communication program promotes sign language and the manual spelling of words by finger movements (finger spelling) as the only approach to communicating with others.

Schools with a strictly manual orientation don't insist that their students wear hearing aids. There are very few schools in the country today that are based solely on manual communication.

Total Communication

This approach is a combination of the oral and manual approaches. Children in total communication programs are encouraged to speechread and to wear hearing aids. They also learn sign language and the manual alphabet so that they can produce words by means of finger spelling or signing.

Cued Speech

Cued speech is the use of hand signals to supply any information that was missed in speechreading. Some people call it a system of communication, while others consider it an adjunct, or visual augmentation, to speech.

What Parents Can Do

Because parents know they should get their child into a language learning program as soon as possible, they usually select the educational approach suggested by the child's diagnostic team. Often, the consulting audiologist or diagnostic center may recommend an educational program that is in the same community or close to the family's home. But this may not necessarily be the best one for the child. Ideally, parents should visit a variety of programs to learn about other philosophies of education and see how they work. By understanding the different approaches, parents may feel more certain that they have selected a course that is right for their child as well as for the family.

Sign Language

Sign language uses both hand and body signs to convey information and to communicate. Among normal-hearing people who have little contact with the deaf, it is commonly thought that sign language is a universal way of communicating—understood by all who use it. But this is not the case.

American Sign Language (ASL) is widely used by deaf people in the United States. It has its own vocabulary, grammar, and syntax, but is only one form of sign language among many. Some other sign language systems are Seeing Essential English (SEE) and Language of Visual Expression (LOVE). These sign systems evolved in an attempt to create a single English language–based sign system, which never happened.

American Sign Language is *not* the same as English, nor does it follow any of the semantics or structure that apply to English. ASL's vocabulary has been estimated to contain about 6,000 signs. English, on the other hand, contains many times this number.

In fact, the relationship between parent and child should take precedence over any advice offered by the experts. If someone insists, for example, that you should use sign language with your deaf child, and you aren't comfortable with this approach, look for another method. Some experts may tell you that once you select an educational program, the child should stay with it despite difficulties. Others call for more flexibility, noting that when a child isn't doing well in a certain program, then it's best to seek another educational approach. As a parent, you are free to disagree and follow your own instincts and preferences.

Two organizations are helpful for parents seeking guidance. The Alexander Graham Bell Association for the Deaf, Inc., offers information on oral speech skills and programs, and the National Association of the Deaf has information available on manual skills and programs.

Another resource for parents of hearing-impaired infants is the John Tracy Clinic. Unlike the other two organizations, which provide information, the John Tracy Clinic takes practical action to encourage parents to become actively involved in the education of their deaf child. The clinic offers free correspondence courses for parents that provide suggestions and instructions on how you can help your child communicate better.

Parents seeking information on cued speech can contact the Cued Speech National Center. Additional information is available from information clearinghouses such as the National Information Center on Deafness. *The addresses of these and other organizations are listed in appendix C.*

Higher Education and Employment Opportunities

Hearing-impaired students who are qualified have a choice of more than 150 postsecondary school programs that are accessible to deaf students. Among these are vocational and technical programs, community colleges, four-year colleges, and universities.

Gallaudet University, in Washington, DC, is the only liberal arts college for the deaf in the world. Undergraduates and those who have completed master's degrees at Gallaudet have gone on to a wide range of professional careers.

The National Technical Institute for the Deaf (NTID), located in Rochester, New York, offers education and training in four broad areas: business, applied science/allied health, engineering technologies, and visual communications. Students may choose to obtain a certificate or associate's degree, or they may enroll in advanced degree programs at the Rochester Institute of Technology.

NTID was created by Congress and receives most of its funds from the U.S. Department of Education. Operating within NTID is the National Center on Employment of the Deaf (NCED), which serves as a placement office for students seeking employment. The NCED office has helped NTID to achieve an enviable average placement rate of 95 percent.

This office also offers orientation and training programs for supervisors and managers who will be working with the deaf employee. Among the topics covered in this half-day workshop are communication, understanding deafness, accommodating the deaf employee, and sensitivity training.

In addition to Gallaudet and NTID, there are a number of regional programs that serve the higher educational needs of hearing-impaired students. They are: California State University, Northridge; Seattle

Community College; St. Paul Technical School, St. Paul, Minnesota; and the University of Tennessee, Knoxville.

NTID is unique in that it calculates its statistics on employment in the same manner as the U.S. Department of Labor's Bureau of Labor Statistics. Other schools that educate the deaf and hard-of-hearing are unlikely to track the placement data on their graduates in the same way, but that doesn't mean that these other programs are less successful. All schools that serve deaf students can help employers recruit qualified employees from their student and graduate rosters.

Finding a Job

In the past, deaf people were underemployed—a problem that the federal government once called the "most serious occupational result of profound deafness." Today, thanks to improvements in educational opportunities and the creation of laws prohibiting discrimination, deaf people are beginning to join the ranks of many professions, including science, architecture, the law, engineering, computer analysis, graphic arts, and manufacturing technology.

The passage of the Americans with Disabilities Act (ADA) of 1990 also has helped bring more deaf people into the workplace. ADA guarantees people with disabilities equal opportunities in employment, public accommodations, transportation, state and local government services, and telecommunications. Thanks to the growing sensitivity to the needs of deaf people, employers have begun to recruit a growing number of qualified deaf workers.

VOCATIONAL TRAINING

Every state has a vocational rehabilitation agency that helps people with disabilities obtain the appropriate training in order to obtain or keep a job.

The vocational rehabilitation (VR) agency in each state is usually listed under the state government section in the telephone book. When you contact this office, ask for an application form. After you complete the form, a VR representative will contact you to set up an interview.

If the VR representative thinks that you may be eligible for the training program, he or she will arrange appointments for medical and

Safety on the Job: Working with the Deaf

Studies have shown that deaf employees have higher-than-average safety records because they have been trained to be more alert to visual signs of trouble than people who depend on sound alone. As a result, deaf employees don't need to have their work environment modified a great deal, although there are some changes that are recommended by the National Center on Employment of the Deaf, including:

- The incorporation of signaling devices into existing alarm systems
- Keeping background noise and vibration in the work area to a minimum, because both can distort sound as received by a hearing aid
- In cases where the deaf employee must wear a pager, the choice of a tactile or vibrating pager so that he or she can respond promptly
- Visual clues to enhance communication, which may mean arranging seats in a circle or semicircle during a meeting or presentation. Another strategy would be the use of visual materials more often during meetings.

When deaf workers communicate by telephone, they may need special equipment, such as an amplifier, a visual alerting signal that flashes when the phone rings, a modified telephone bell, a computer modem, or a telecommunications device for the deaf (TDD). In some situations, such as a staff meeting, sales conference, or annual meeting, a deaf employee may prefer to have an interpreter available to ensure that all of the communication is received.

The NCED also stresses the importance of including the deaf employee in the company's social activities, such as coffee breaks, lunch gatherings, and office parties.

hearing tests. Aptitude and psychological tests also may be ordered. After completion of the tests and evaluation of the results, the VR counselor will determine whether you qualify for vocational rehabilitation services.

The services may be as simple as offering you assistance in obtaining a hearing aid or assistive listening device. Or your counselor may determine that you need to explore various career options or pursue needed training.

10

Choosing and Paying for Hearing Health Care

Admitting to a hearing problem is a major step for many people. Knowing which providers of hearing health care to seek out makes it easier to get the help you need. Trying to fix a hearing problem on your own—such as buying a hearing aid without a medical evaluation—is an open invitation to frustration and dissatisfaction. Instead, you should first consult a physician so that any medically correctable cause of your hearing loss can be ruled out.

CHOOSING A HEARING SPECIALIST

There are many professionals who can determine whether you have a hearing loss and will work with you to repair or correct the problem:

- otolaryngologists, also called ear, nose, and throat (ENT) physicians
- audiologists
- speech-language pathologists

- hearing aid dispensers
- teachers of the deaf
- vocational and rehabilitation counselors

Otolaryngologists

In the past, otolaryngologists were called ear, nose, and throat (ENT) doctors, but more recently this area has come to include the related structures of the head and neck. Many subspecialties also exist within the field of otolaryngology, including physicians who specialize in the diagnosis and treatment of

- problems of the ear (otology)
- problems of the nose and sinuses (rhinology)
- allergic disorders (otolaryngic allergy)
- neurological ear problems (neurotology)
- problems of the larynx, including voice disorders (laryngology)
- disorders of the esophagus (bronchoesophagology)
- benign and malignant tumors of the head and neck (head and neck oncology)
- vestibular/balance disorders (neurotology)
- taste and smell disorders
- reconstructive surgery of the ear, nose, throat, and related structures of the head and neck (facial, plastic, and reconstructive surgery)
- children's ear, nose, and throat disorders (pediatric otolaryngology)

All otolaryngologists, no matter their specialty, are qualified to perform examinations relating to these specific areas. Some prefer to use a subspecialty title, while others, even if they have a special interest in a particular area, simply designate themselves as otolaryngologists.

Qualifications. To qualify as a specialist in otolaryngology–head and neck surgery, a graduate of a medical school must enter a medical residency program at an approved teaching hospital. The residency program of study and training lasts five years. Some doctors may also take fellowship training, which entails additional study or research after completing their residency requirements.

In order to obtain board certification from the American Board of Otolaryngology, a physician must successfully complete an approved residency program and then pass examinations given in a specialty area of medical and surgical expertise. When a doctor is a board-certified specialist or subspecialist in otolaryngology, it means that he or she is qualified to practice in the field.

Some specialists may call themselves board-eligible and retain that status throughout their careers simply because the medical system allows it. A board-eligible physician is one who has completed the required training for a specialty but either has never taken or has failed the board examinations. In checking the credentials of a board-eligible doctor, you have the right to ask why this physician is listed as a specialist but has not yet become board-certified.

To verify the training and credentials of an otolaryngologist, consult the *Directory of Medical Specialists* in the reference section of your public library. Unfortunately, some specialists with excellent credentials may choose to list neither their names nor their biographies in this directory.

In addition to board certification, all states require that each physician obtain a state license in order to practice.

How to find an otolaryngologist. If you need the services of an otolaryngologist, ask your family physician to recommend a few specialists. If you don't have a personal physician, call the department of otolaryngology at the nearest university medical school. Or call the medical center nearest to you for the names of some hearing specialists on their staff.

The American Academy of Otolaryngology—Head and Neck Surgery also provides the names of otolaryngologists. The academy will send you a list of board-certified otolaryngologists in your zip code area, metropolitan area, or state, depending on where you live. (For the academy's address, consult appendix C.)

The first visit. If you are seeing an otolaryngologist for the first time, ask the following questions:

- *What is your fee?* Also inquire about any additional charges. Ask whether or not the doctor will accept your insurance as payment, or if payment is required before or immediately after consultation and/or treatment.
- *What is your hospital affiliation?* Inquire if the otolaryngologist's hospital or medical center provides the best setting and staff for any surgical treatment needed.

- *How often do you perform the procedure, treatment, or surgery that you have recommended?* Don't be reluctant to ask about the surgery, what success rate the doctor has had with a particular procedure, and how it compares with national figures. Also question him or her about the possibility of complications. When a specialist downplays the need for this information, find another specialist.
- *If I require surgery, will you be performing the operation yourself?* When a procedure takes place at a teaching hospital, a resident in training may perform the surgery under the supervision of an attending specialist. If your otolaryngologist explains that a resident will do all or part of the procedure, you have the right to request—and insist—that the doctor you are paying for performs the operation.

After a physical examination and some office tests, the otolaryngologist may be able to determine the cause of your hearing loss, based on observation. For example, your hearing problem may be due to excess earwax, which the physician can then remove. More often, the cause of hearing loss is not as easily resolved. Depending on your diagnosis, the otolaryngologist may prescribe medication or surgery.

If the otolaryngologist cannot diagnose your problem from information gleaned during the examination and office testing, additional hearing tests will be prescribed. These tests are administered by an audiologist (see chapter 3).

The Audiologist

An audiologist is a health-care professional who identifies and measures hearing loss and helps to rehabilitate people with hearing disorders.

Audiologists may work as private practitioners, or they may be associated with an otolaryngology practice. These professionals are also found in medical centers, hospitals, universities, and speech-hearing centers. Still others work in private industry, where they may be involved in the testing and assessment of workers and in hearing-conversation programs. Audiologists serve as consultants for noise abatement agencies, and in the research and development of new audiological testing methods and hearing devices.

Prevention of hearing loss is a special interest for some audiologists, particularly those who work in industry and research settings. Rehabilitation services, such as prescribing and dispensing hearing aids, may be the area of specialization for others.

Qualifications. The minimum level of education necessary to become an accredited audiologist is a master's degree. This educational standard was established by the American Speech-Language-Hearing Association (ASHA), a national organization that awards the only professional credentials for audiologists that are fully recognized in every state.

Students who decide they want to pursue a career in audiology are advised by ASHA to select an undergraduate college or university that will provide them with a strong background in liberal arts and sciences. Many undergraduate programs also offer courses that deal with communication sciences and hearing disorders.

Approximately 260 academic programs in the United States and Canada now offer a master's degree in audiology and speech-language pathology. Of these, about 100 programs focus on audiology alone. About two-thirds of these programs have been accredited by ASHA in audiology and speech-language. Doctorate-level programs also are available.

The letters CCC (for Certificate of Clinical Competence) follow the names of qualified audiologists and speech-language pathologists, and CCC-A indicates certification in the field of audiology. A certified professional has completed the training required for a master's degree, has had 350 hours of supervised clinical experience, and has also passed a written examination.

Certification is voluntary, but many medical centers, hospitals, clinics, and other facilities now require it. Today, most states have laws requiring an audiologist to be licensed in order to practice. Medicare and Medicaid will not reimburse private practitioners in this field for services to patients unless the professional holds either a license or the CCC.

In 1988 the American Academy of Audiology (AAA) was established as a professional association for audiologists. Academy members must hold the CCC-A certification or have at least a master's degree in audiology, and they must be licensed by their state to practice audiology. The academy also is working toward the establishment of professional doctoral degree programs at universities nationwide that would offer the Au.D. degree.

How to find an audiologist. If you already have been to an otolaryngologist, and he or she has ordered hearing tests, your introduction to this professional may be as simple as walking down the hall. If you are seeking an outside audiologist, ASHA is an excellent source of information. When you call or write this organization (see appendix C), you will receive a list of professionals and/or programs in your state.

The American Academy of Audiology also can provide information. If you would like a list of qualified audiologists in your geographical area, contact this organization.

If there is a college or university in your town, call and ask if there is a speech clinic associated with the school. This facility may provide the services you need. Many hospitals also offer services related to hearing or speech language disorders.

The Yellow Pages of your telephone directory also list audiologists for each telephone service area. If the qualified audiologist you first contact cannot provide the kind of service you need, he or she may be able to point you in the right direction.

If you are seeking audiological services for a child, call the school district superintendent's office or the special education division. By asking questions and seeking additional information, you should be able to get help for your child.

Questions to ask. Before undergoing any evaluations, ask an audiologist or speech-language professional the following questions:

- Are you certified and/or licensed?
- What age groups do you work with?
- Do you work primarily with a particular speech, language, or hearing disorder? If so, which one?
- How soon can I be seen for an evaluation?
- Once I am evaluated, is there a waiting list for treatment? If so, how long is it?
- If you cannot work with me, whom would you recommend in your place?
- Do I need to be referred to your clinic by a particular source such as a community agency?
- Once I have been evaluated, will you be able to anticipate the amount of time needed to correct my problem?
- Do you dispense/sell hearing aids? If not, will you help me get one from another source?

- Do you provide auditory training, speechreading, and/or hearing aid orientation for the new hearing aid user?
- Do you provide day classes for children with language disorders?
- How much do you charge?
- What sources of third-party payment may be available to me?

Speech-Language Pathologists

Speech-language pathologists are professionals who are trained to identify specific problems in oral communication. They can determine the severity of the problem and provide nonmedical therapy.

These health-care providers work in a variety of settings, including schools or preschool programs. Others are found in hospitals, where they work with children who have speech disorders as the result of an anatomical problem, such as a cleft palate.

Many adults also require the services of a speech-language pathologist. People who have suffered a stroke may need professional help in regaining the use of language, for example. Those who stutter, have problems with their voice and articulation, or want to modify a regional accent would consult a speech-language pathologist. Because hearing loss affects the quality of speech, these experts also work with hard-of-hearing people who don't want to lose their speaking skills.

Qualifications. Speech-language pathologists must meet the same educational and professional standards as audiologists.

How to find a speech-language pathologist. If you, your child, or someone you know has a communications disorder that calls for the services of a team of specialists, then your otolaryngologist or audiologist may call in or refer you to a speech-language pathologist. But if you are searching for one on your own, you can contact ASHA and request a list of accredited professionals who practice in your area (see appendix C).

Speech-language pathologists also may be found at colleges, universities, teaching hospitals, rehabilitation centers, skilled-nursing facilities, health departments, and schools. Other sources include the Yellow Pages of your telephone book under the heading "Speech and Language Pathologists."

Ask the same questions of a speech-language pathologist as you would an audiologist.

Hearing Aid Dispensers

Dispensers sell and service hearing aids. Although they must have some training in the measurement and interpretation of hearing tests, they are not required to have a college degree. Some dispensers, however, obtain certification from the National Board for Certification of Hearing Instrument Sciences, indicated by the letters *BC-HIS*. The International Hearing Society is the professional group that oversees this board. In order to be certified, dispensers must attend continuing education courses and successfully pass a national examination.

Teachers of the Deaf

A teacher of the deaf is a nonmedical, specially trained educator who may instruct a hearing-impaired child through manual communication, total communication, an oral approach, or cued speech.

Because deafness is now identified earlier in childhood, an educator of the deaf often can be found working with an audiologist and a speech-language pathologist during a child's preschool years.

Vocational and Rehabilitation Counselors

Each state's vocational rehabilitation (VR) agency employs specially trained caseworkers whose primary job is to help people with disabilities—including those who are hearing-impaired—either to keep their present jobs or get retraining for new ones.

These caseworkers are counselors who first must determine one's eligibility for services. If the counselor considers you an appropriate candidate based on your written application and personal screening interview, you are eligible to receive medical, hearing, and vocational evaluations. Your VR counselor will meet with you to discuss a plan for achieving your goals. Once the plan has been drawn up, the VR counselor may offer you either counseling, guidance, or training services.

Depending on your need, motivation, and attitude, the services may be simple or more far-reaching. In some cases, the counselor may decide that you would benefit from having an assistive listening device for your workplace. Or the counselor may help you explore a variety of occupational possibilities and training.

If you disagree with a decision made by a VR counselor, you have the right to file an appeal with the agency and request that the VR administration review the decision. VR clients have certain rights that allow their full participation in the rehabilitation process.

Other types of counselors also work in the rehabilitation of adults and children with a hearing impairment. Depending on the program, your counselor may be an audiologist, a speech-language pathologist, a physician, a medical social worker, a public health nurse, or an educator of the hearing-impaired.

Counselors may be responsible for a number of concerns: interpreting information given by the specialists you are working with, explaining insurance regulations that apply to your therapy, helping you resolve or get information about help for financial problems, and encouraging your active participation in your rehabilitation.

PAYING FOR HEARING HEALTH-CARE SERVICES

Cost is always a major concern for most people with hearing loss. Most private and public insurance plans provide coverage for the medical and surgical treatment of a hearing problem. But only 5 to 10 percent of hearing loss can be corrected medically or surgically.

Unfortunately, many hearing-impaired people who don't need medical treatment but who would benefit from wearing a hearing aid can't expect any help from their insurance carrier. This population includes men and women age 65 and older who participate in Medicare, the federal health insurance program. Medicare, along with many private insurers, will not pay for a hearing aid or listening device.

In most cases, when audiological testing services are required in order to make a diagnosis of a medical or surgical hearing problem, these services are usually covered. But if you suffer from gradual hearing loss, go for a medical examination and hearing test by an audiologist, and find that all you need is a hearing aid, your insurer may not even cover the testing.

It's a good idea to find out exactly what services are covered by your insurance and whether you'll be expected to pay part or all of your bill up front when you visit a hearing specialist. Even if most charges are covered, you still may be required to pay a deductible or make a copayment, depending on your particular health-care plan.

TYPES OF INSURANCE COVERAGE

There are two basic kinds of insurance—government or private. Governmental insurance includes Medicare (the federal program) and Medicaid (which is administered by each state). Private insurance includes traditional health plans offered by commercial insurance companies, as well as those of health maintenance organizations (HMOs), preferred provider organizations (PPOs), and plans that are funded by the employers themselves.

The following is a general idea of what kind of insurance coverage you can expect for hearing problems.

Governmental Insurance Programs

Medicare. Medicare was designed to provide federal health insurance coverage to people over 65 years old and to those who are under 65 but disabled. Your eligibility for Medicare is not based on your income or financial assets. If you have a diagnosed condition such as otosclerosis, a medically correctable disorder of the middle ear, Medicare would cover the cost of your examination, diagnostic hearing tests, and any possible surgery.

When it comes to hearing services, Medicare's coverage is extremely limited. The program will not pay for a hearing aid or anything related to it, including examinations and audiological testing.

According to the criteria for Medicare coverage, audiological evaluations are covered only when a physician orders testing to help diagnose a hearing loss or a related medical problem. Under Medicare's coverage guidelines, the federal insurer will cover therapeutic services provided by an audiologist only if a physician has ordered the service and if the audiologist is under the direct supervision of a physician on the premises.

Medicare does cover cochlear implants, but the amount of reimbursement that the federal insurer provides to participating hospitals and medical centers for this procedure is very low. Some service organizations, such as Lions Clubs, have been willing to help underwrite some of the rehabilitation costs, however.

A person who receives a cochlear implant requires several months of special training or rehabilitation in how to use the device effectively. In the past, rehabilitation was not a service that routinely qualified for reimbursement. The Health Care Financing Administration has now issued a policy that directs Medicare insurance carriers nationwide to pay for the rehabilitation costs of cochlear implant patients for one year.

Beware of False Advertising

In 1993 seven hearing aid dealers in different areas of the United States agreed to correct advertising that the federal government said misled elderly customers about Medicare reimbursement. The advertisements contained such phrases as "sales and service . . . all major brands . . . Medicare welcome." The dealers had to change misleading information in phone books and were enjoined against giving similar inaccurate information to customers, upon penalty of a $10,000 fine.

Medicare does not cover the cost of hearing aids and does not reimburse patients for hearing tests conducted for the purpose of prescribing or fitting hearing aids. Medicare covers only hearing tests performed to diagnose medical problems.

Medicaid. Medicaid, the state-run health insurance program, generally serves the aged, blind, disabled, medically needy, and families with dependent children. Each state has a different income requirement that must be met in order to qualify for Medicaid. Eligibility is contingent on meeting a strict low-income standard.

Children who are eligible for Medicaid can participate in a program that exists in practically every state: Early and Periodic Screening Diagnosis and Treatment (EPSDT). Under this program, children are eligible for audiology services and a hearing aid.

The upper-age requirements for EPSDT may not be the same in each state. If you think your child may be eligible for hearing healthcare benefits under this program, contact your local Medicaid office.

Coverage varies from state to state for adults who qualify for Medicaid. About half the states cover essentials like audiology services and offer some reimbursement to providers for hearing aids.

Private Insurance Programs

Indemnity plans. Indemnity plans, sometimes called fee-for-service insurance, allow you to choose your own doctor or qualified provider, and the insurance company will pay for all or part of your treatment.

Your insurance carrier's payment usually will be based on usual, customary, and reasonable (UCR) fees charged by hearing health-care providers in your geographic area. Some plans may require that you get prior approval from the company before you see a doctor or audiologist for services.

(Medicare is adopting new payment guidelines that are expected to be phased in by 1996. Private insurance carriers most likely will follow Medicare's lead in changing the rules that govern payments to physicians and providers, so you can expect that reimbursement to your providers will change as well.)

Most of these plans will cover a visit to a licensed otolaryngologist for a medical examination. If the physician orders diagnostic hearing tests by an audiologist, these services are likely to be covered, too. But be sure you review your insurance policy before getting the tests. Some plans clearly state that they will not cover audiology services unless they are rendered in a hospital setting.

Health maintenance organizations. Health maintenance organizations (HMOs) are prepaid insurance plans in which you pay a set annual fee in advance that entitles you to medical, surgical, and hospital care. Once you are a member, instead of paying a deductible, you pay a small fee each time you visit a doctor.

There are different types of HMOs. A staff HMO has its doctors, specialists, nurses, and other staff members in a single setting. Depending on the size of this HMO model, there is likely to be an otolaryngologist and an audiologist on staff. If you belong to a smaller HMO, check your benefits booklet to determine whether hearing health-care services and hearing aids are covered.

HMO coverage requires that you obtain any necessary medical, diagnostic, and rehabilitation services from providers who have been approved by the HMO. Your primary care physician must authorize any services before you receive them. Check with your HMO office before seeking out any hearing health-care services.

HMOs have more of an incentive to keep the costs of medical care down than do traditional insurance plans: They cannot make a profit unless costs are kept below the amount of per capita prepaid enrollments per year. If an HMO pays out more in costs than it brings in, it operates at a loss.

With this in mind, HMOs may be less willing to cover the expense of a high-priced treatment such as a cochlear implant. This treatment, which is approved by the FDA, is a very costly therapy and involves a period of rehabilitation after the surgery. If you or someone in your family is a potential candidate for a cochlear implant, be certain to check your HMO policy or booklet to see if you are covered.

Preferred provider organizations. Preferred provider organizations (PPOs) are yet another alternative to traditional health insurance plans. Under this kind of arrangement, physicians, hospitals, and other providers arrange with employers to offer prepaid discounted coverage for their employees' medical care.

The PPO system usually doesn't require a deductible, although you can expect to pay a small fee for an office visit. But if you seek medical care from a provider who isn't under contract with the PPO, you will have to pay more of the fee.

Although this kind of coverage was designed with cost containment in mind, it may not be as restrictive as some HMOs in terms of offering certain services—such as hearing health care. Once again, read your health-care benefits plan to determine whether hearing services are covered.

Self-insured plans. When a company offers *self-insurance* to its employees in place of traditional insurance, it means that the company itself assumes the financial risk when claims are made. The plan managers usually invest the insurance fund's money until they need to tap the fund to make payments on claims.

A growing number of companies are choosing self-funded insurance plans, mainly because they can design the plans themselves and decide what should be covered and what can be excluded. Self-insured plans are exempt from paying any costly state-mandated benefits and also receive an exemption from state taxes on insurance premiums.

Because hearing loss or deafness is not a life-threatening illness, some employers may decide not to cover these disorders by excluding benefits for hearing tests, hearing aids, or cochlear implants.

Tips on Obtaining Health-Care Benefits

Be sure to look at a description of your benefits plan before you go to an audiologist for hearing tests—especially if your coverage is an indemnity or a self-insured company plan. If the language is unclear and you're not certain whether coverage is provided or not, call the health plan's representative to check.

Write down the name of the person you speak with and take notes so that you have a record of the conversation. If the representative tells you to go ahead and get the hearing evaluation because the plan will cover it, then you should feel secure with that clearance. If the provider presents the bill to the company and it refuses to pay, you can pull out your notes from your earlier inquiry and tell the provider to speak with the company's representative.

REHABILITATION THERAPY

When illness or injury affects your hearing and your ability to speak, your doctor may order rehabilitation therapy to help restore your speech-language capability. Depending on the proposed period of rehabilitation and the nature of your disorder, your insurance plan may offer coverage, deny it, or be open to negotiating with you. In most cases, getting your plan to pay for rehabilitation can be difficult: Insurance companies don't like to pay for long-term services.

If you know that the rehabilitation schedule will last for a definite number of weeks or months and that it is expected to return you to a productive life, let your insurer know. Explain what each session of rehabilitation will entail and that it's not an open-ended arrangement, but one that will operate under a certain schedule for a limited period of time.

Your audiologist or speech-language pathologist can tell you how long your rehabilitation should last and also be able to give your insurer an idea of how much it will cost. These professionals often serve as advocates for patients who are seeking insurance coverage for rehabilitation services.

Your insurer may be willing to work with you in allowing rehabilitation coverage, or you may be turned down altogether. In either case, it's worth the try. The number of people eligible for hearing benefits is increasing. The growth in coverage for hearing problems, however, lags far behind the greater demand for dental and vision benefits. Many companies include hearing benefits in their health-care plans, but often write restrictions and exclusions into them. Again, negotiations with an employer are worth trying.

Talk to Your Employer

If you and your coworkers would like to have hearing health-care benefits as part of your insurance plan, ASHA recommends the following steps:

- Talk with a representative from your benefits office or personnel office. Let them know that you would like coverage for hearing and speech-language services included in your benefits plan.
- Tell your coworkers why this kind of coverage is important. Ask them to stop by the company's benefits office and request coverage.
- If you are a member of a labor union, talk with union leaders and ask them to work for getting a hearing-care benefit.

ASHA works with employees and benefits administrators who are interested in developing a hearing benefits program. For more information, contact ASHA (see appendix C).

FUNDING SOURCES

If you or someone you know can't afford to pay for a hearing aid or assistive listening device, there are programs and organizations that can help. Finding out what help is available and knowing where to look for it is much of the battle. Unfortunately, there is no single source of information about the vast patchwork of outside funding that exists nationwide.

Here are a number of programs, organizations, and agencies that can assist you in your search.

- *Purchase programs.* If it is determined that you would benefit from a hearing aid and this service isn't covered by insurance (and you don't qualify for government-sponsored or other benefits), don't despair. You may have to pay out of pocket, but if you explain your financial situation to your audiologist, he or she may be able to help you. Many audiologists offer a purchase program plan, which allows you to pay off the cost of the hearing aid over a period of time.
- *Civic organizations.* Civic and service organizations often are potential sources of help for people needing hearing aids. Because the service projects undertaken by these groups vary in each community, it is recommended that you check with the local chapters of these organizations for information.

  One program that is offered by various local chapters of the Lions Club International is the Lions Club Equipment Purchase Assistance. This program provides telecommunications devices for the deaf (TDDs) and hearing-ear dogs (see box) for people who request them. The national headquarters of the Lions Club does not keep track of the assistance offered by each of its local chapters, however. In order to learn whether a chapter near you provides or would consider providing equipment-purchase assistance to the hearing-impaired, contact your local Lions Club.
- *Local agencies.* In many areas, there are United Way Speech and Hearing Centers that may be able to provide hearing aids or assistive listening devices at a lower price. Some other possible sources of help would include organizations such as the New York League for the Hard-of-Hearing, the Chicago Hearing Aid Society, and similar centers in other cities.
- *State agencies and programs.* If you don't meet the eligibility requirements for Medicaid, but can't afford to buy a hearing aid, you might consider looking into other state programs to see if help is available. One place to check is your state commission for deaf and hard-of-hearing people.
- *Veterans Administration programs.* Veterans who have acquired a hearing loss while serving in the military, or whose service-related injury led to a later hearing impairment, may be eligible for assistance from the Department of Veterans Affairs. Each decision for assistance is made on a case-by-case basis following a hearing evaluation conducted by a VA audiologist. (For more

The Hearing-Ear Dog Program

In 1976 the American Humane Association in Denver began training dogs to react to specific sounds in order to meet the needs of the hearing-impaired. The demand for these dogs grew beyond the limits of a single facility, and now hearing-dog training centers can be found in various parts of the United States.

The hearing-ear dog programs usually give priority to severely or profoundly deaf adults. A preplacement visit to the center assesses applicants' need for a hearing-ear dog, their commitment to meeting the animal's needs, and their determination to reinforce the response training. Each dog is chosen specifically for its deaf master. During the training period, recipients are encouraged to stay in close contact with the Hearing Dog Center to maintain an active interest in their dog's progress.

Hearing-ear dogs are trained to respond to certain sounds by making physical contact with the owner and leading him or her to the source of the sound. Training takes about four months to complete. A placement counselor takes the dog to its new home for a final week of training to ensure a smooth transition.

Every effort is made to accommodate the cost of the dog and its training to the recipient's resources. This includes helping the deaf person find financial sponsors for the dog. No applicants are denied a hearing dog because of their inability to pay.

For further information, contact:

The Hearing Dog Resource Center
P.O. Box 1080
Renton, WA 98057-1080
(206) 226-7357 (8:30 A.M.–5 P.M. Pacific standard time)
(206) 235-3179 (Voice and TDD)

information on the VA Hearing Aid Program, see chapter 4. Consult appendix A for the latest VA evaluations of hearing aids.)

- *Hearing aid banks.* Operated by a nonprofit organization called Hear Now, the National Hearing Aid Bank in Denver supplies donated new, used, and reconditioned hearing aids. It also provides help with cochlear implants for qualified applicants.

Hear Now also requests hearing-care providers, manufacturers, and community service groups to volunteer their time, products, and funds to help people who are deaf and hard-of-hearing (see appendix C).

- *Vocational rehabilitation programs.* State vocational rehabilitation (VR) programs are based on certain standards and policies established by the federal Rehabilitation Services Administration, a division of the Department of Education. Funding for VR programs comes from federal and state budgets.

  Because each state is allowed to administer its own program, there is room for some flexibility in determining eligibility and the scope of services. Assistance may include financial assistance in the purchase of a hearing aid or assistive listening device, or for education and training. It may also include help with job placement.

  To locate the VR office in your state, look in the Yellow Pages under the state government listings for "Vocational Rehabilitation" or "Rehabilitation." In some states, this office may fall under another department's jurisdiction, such as labor or education.
- *Technology-related assistance.* The Technology-Related Assistance for Individuals with Disabilities Act of 1988 established a program of grants to states for people with disabilities.

  Each state develops its own program and includes vocational rehabilitation agencies, human resource agencies, universities, and rehabilitation technology centers. More than half of all states have already received funding for this program. By 1995, all states are expected to have this program fully funded and in place.

  Among the assistive devices that may be available for qualified state residents are telecommunications devices for the deaf (TDDs), telecaption decoders, and safety devices. For the address, telephone number, and name of the person you should contact in your state, write or call: RESNA Technical Assistance Project, 1101 Connecticut Avenue N.W., Suite 700, Washington, DC 20036. Telephone: (202) 857-1140 (Voice and TDD).
- *TDD programs.* Some states have programs that provide telecommunications devices for the deaf (TDDs) to all deaf and hard-of-hearing people. In addition to TDDs, the states may provide

telephone signaling devices and amplifiers as well as the training to operate them.

For information, check with your telephone company, state council or commission for the hearing-impaired, bureau of vocational rehabilitation, or department of human services.

- *Low-interest or no-interest loans.* Loans that either carry very low interest or are interest-free are available in some states for the purchase of assistive hearing devices. Check with your state to see if there are any restrictions tied to these loans.

  Pennsylvania and New York offer residents low-interest loans, and Minnesota provides no-interest loans. Residents of western Kentucky, southwestern Indiana, and southeastern Illinois can apply for loans through the Deaf Social Service Agency for the Tri-State Area in Evansville, Illinois.
- *Self-help groups.* If you are a deaf adult, the national organization Self-Help for Hard-of-Hearing People (SHHH) promotes awareness of information about products, services, and possible sources of help (see appendix C).

GLOSSARY

Acoustic neuroma. A benign growth on the vestibular nerves, the nerves that run from the inner ear to the brain stem. Named acoustic neuroma because hearing loss is an early symptom.

Acute otitis media. An infection of the middle ear.

Aerotitis (barotrauma). Temporary injury of the middle ear—usually causing pain and decreased hearing. It is due to failure to equalize pressure in the middle ear during plane flights.

Analog hearing aid. A hearing device that works with sound as frequencies; a conventional hearing aid that receives sound and amplifies it.

ASHA. American Speech-Language-Hearing Association.

Assistive listening devices (ALDs). Amplifying devices for the home and office that can help the hearing-impaired person.

Audiogram. A hearing test.

Audiologist. A professional who specializes in testing hearing function.

Audio loop. An assistive listening device: A microphone and an amplifier are attached to a wire that circles the listening area. Persons with a T-coil on their hearing aid or headset can pick up the sound as if the speaker was sitting next to them.

Auditory (acoustic) nerve. The nerve that carries sound from the inner ear to the brain.

Aural atresia. Underdeveloped ears. This condition can involve the outer, middle, and inner ear.

Auricle. The outer part of the ear.

Barotrauma. *See* Aerotitis.

Behind-the-ear (BTE) hearing aid. A hearing device with the microphone and amplifier located in a case behind the ear.

Bell's palsy. A facial paralysis that occurs without a known cause.

BICROS hearing aid. Technically, a bilateral contralateral routing of signals. BICROS hearing aids are useful when hearing in the "good" ear is also impaired and needs amplification.

Cerumen. Earwax.

Cholesteatoma. A skin cyst in the middle ear.

Cochlea. A snail-shaped structure in the inner ear that houses the hearing organ.

Cochlear implants. Electronic devices that are implanted in the inner ear and enable a deaf person to hear.

Compression circuits. Allows control of the sound that a hearing aid amplifies, so that loud sounds are amplified less than quiet sounds.

Conductive hearing loss. Hearing loss due to a problem in the outer and middle ear that prevents sound from getting to the inner ear.

CROS hearing aid. A hearing aid that sends the sound from one ear into the other ear (useful when one ear does not hear).

Deaf. A hearing impairment so severe that a person cannot process any sound information.

Decibels. A system of rating the loudness of sound. The larger the number, the louder the sound.

Digital hearing aid. A hearing aid that converts sounds to numerical values. These values can then be altered to amplify the sounds differentially.

Digitally controlled hearing aid. A hearing device that receives sounds, codes them numerically (digitally), modifies them, and then plays them back louder.

Eardrum. A membrane that forms a tight seal between the outer ear and the middle ear. The vibrating eardrum transmits the waves of sound to the bones in the middle ear.

Electronystagmography (ENG). A series of tests designed to explore the function of the balance system.

Endolymph. A fluid, found in the inner ear, that has a high potassium content.

Eustachian tube. A tube connecting the middle ear and the back of the nose. It allows air to enter the middle ear.

Evoked response audiometry (ERA). A test to measure the transmission of sound from the ear to the brain.

Exostosis. Bony growths in the ear canal, usually from cold-water swimming.

External otitis. Swimmer's ear, which is an infection in the ear canal.

Facial nerve. Nerve that controls the movement of muscles that allow facial expressions. Because the facial nerve runs through the ear, an ailment that affects the ear can also interfere with the nerve, resulting in a facial paralysis, such as Bell's palsy.

Frequency. The vibrating speed of sound waves. Frequency determines whether the pitch is high (high frequency) or low (low frequency).

Frequency range. The high and low tones that are amplified by a hearing aid.

Frequency response. The gain that a hearing aid has across different frequencies.

Gain. The number of decibels that a hearing aid can amplify.

Hair cells. Special sensory cells in the inner ear that respond to specific learning tones.

Hard-of-hearing. People who have trouble hearing but can benefit from some form of amplification.

Hearing-impaired. Hearing that is not in the normal range. The hearing loss can be mild to severe to profound.

Hertz (Hz). The frequency of sound waves (cycles per second). The higher the frequency, the higher the tone.

High pass hearing aid. A hearing aid that allows high-frequency speech sounds to be amplified more than low-frequency background noise (see appendix A).

Incus (anvil). The second middle-ear bone.

Infrared system. Sound converts into light. The light reflects around a room and those with receivers pick up the light, which is then converted back into sound.

Infrasound. Sound whose vibrations are so slow (low frequency) that they are below the detection level of the human ear.

Inner ear. Consists of the cochlea (hearing organ) and labyrinth (balance organ).

In-the-canal (ITC) hearing aid. A type of hearing aid that is worn inside the ear canal.

In-the-ear (ITE) hearing aid. A hearing device that is entirely located in the auricle and ear canal.

Labyrinth. An inner-ear structure housing the organs of balance: the utricle, saccule, and semicircular canals.

Labyrinthectomy. A surgical operation, meant to restore balance, that involves destroying inner-ear function. Any remaining hearing is lost in the ear.

Labyrinthitis. An infection of the inner ear causing dizziness and hearing loss.

Malleus (hammer). The first middle-ear bone.

Manual communication training. Educational program using sign language for communication.

Masking. Playing a sound in one ear while testing the opposite ear. Also means substituting music or white sound to cover up tinnitus (noise in the ear).

Mastoid. Bony cavity located behind the ear.

Mastoiditis. An infection in the mastoid.

Ménière's disease. An illness characterized by episodic vertigo, tinnitus, and fluctuating hearing. It is caused by fluid imbalance in the inner ear.

Middle ear. The space between the outer and inner ears, it contains air and the three bones of hearing, or ossicles.

Myringotomy. A drainage cut made in the eardrum.

Nasopharynx. The area behind the nose and above the soft palate.

Nystagmus. Abnormal eye movements: a slow drifting of the eyes to one side followed by a quick recovery to the original line of sight.

Oral communication training. Educational program for the hard-of-hearing, using sounds to teach speech and language.

OSHA. Occupational Safety and Health Administration. A federal agency that oversees safety in the workplace.

Ossicles. The three bones that send sound from the eardrum to the inner ear: malleus (hammer), incus (anvil), and stapes (stirrup).

Otalgia. Ear pain.

Otolaryngologist. Physician who specializes in diagnosing and treating disorders of the ear, nose, and throat.

Otologist. Physician who specializes in diagnosing and treating disorders of the ear.

Otosclerosis. A genetic disorder that causes abnormal bone growth in the ear, resulting in a conductive hearing loss. Sometimes a sensorineural hearing loss occurs, too.

Otoscope. An instrument to examine the ear.

Ototoxic drugs. Drugs that can damage the inner ear, hearing, or balance system.

Outer ear. The auricle, ear canal, and the eardrum.

Output. The loudest sound made by a hearing aid.

Perilymph. A fluid in the inner ear that is similar to spinal fluid.

Perilymph fistula. A leak of fluid from the inner ear to the middle ear.

Posturography. A computerized test of balance function.

Presbycusis. Hearing loss due to aging.

Programmable hearing aid. A hearing aid device that features several channels. These channels can be set for different listening situations to improve hearing.

Proprioception. Muscle and joint messages to the brain, telling it what position they occupy at any given time.

Pure tones. Sounds that are composed of only one frequency.

Real ear measurement. Testing the actual output of the hearing aid at the eardrum.

Recruitment. Perception that loud sounds are too loud. This condition occurs with inner-ear hearing loss.

Saccule. Inner-ear balancing structure that measures linear motion.

Semicircular canals. Inner-ear balancing structure that measures angular motion.

Sensorineural hearing loss. Hearing loss due to a problem in the inner ear, along the auditory nerve, or in the brain.

Serous otitis media. Fluid in the middle ear.

Sign language. A collection of hand and arm signals that convey meaning.

Sociocusis. Hearing loss caused by aging as well as environmental noise at home and in the workplace.

Speechreading. Using both lipreading and other visual clues to improve hearing and understanding.

Speech reception threshold (SRT). The minimum volume at which a person can hear speech.

Stapedectomy. A surgical procedure to correct hearing loss due to otosclerosis.

Stapes (stirrup). The third middle-ear bone.

Telecoil. A circuit in a hearing aid that allows the amplification of a telephone signal with a hearing aid. Also called T-coil.

Telecommunications devices for the deaf (TDDs). Devices that send typewritten messages over the telephone. (Also known as TT.)

Temporal bone. The bone in the skull in which the ear is located.

Temporary threshold shift. A short-term loss of hearing, usually due to loud noise exposure.

Tinnitus. The perception of sound in the ear or head without any external cause.

Tinnitus maskers. Devices that make a noise in the ear to drown out the tinnitus.

Total communication training. Language training that combines oral and manual techniques.

T-switch. The switch on a hearing aid that turns on the telecoil.

Tympanic membrane. Eardrum.

Tympanogram. A test of eardrum motion and middle-ear pressure.

Tympanometry. Testing of eardrum motion and middle-ear pressure.

Tympanoplasty. An operation to repair the eardrum and the ossicles.

Utricle. Inner-ear balancing structure that measures gravity and linear motion.

Ventilation tubes. Tubes placed in the eardrum to drain fluid and allow aeration of the middle ear.

Vertigo. The sensation of motion—either of immediate surroundings or of oneself—when actually there is no motion.

Vestibular nerve. The nerve that carries the balance signals from the inner ear to the brain.

Vestibular neuritis. An inflammation of the inner ear, causing vertigo.

APPENDIX A

Department of Veterans Affairs Review of Hearing Aids, 1992–93

The Department of Veterans Affairs (VA) invited manufacturers to participate in its 1992–93 hearing aid testing program. Fifteen manufacturers submitted 43 stock models—approximately 12 percent of the more than 500 hearing aid models currently available in the United States and abroad.

The VA tests stock models and custom ITE (in-the-ear) aids in alternate years. Stock models including regular, CROS, BICROS (which amplifies sound to the good hearing ear), and High Pass (which contains a filter that helps emphasize high-frequency sounds) were tested in Contract Year 1992. The ones selected by the VA will remain on the VA list for two years. New and improved hearing aids are developed each year, and as a result, the VA contract list varies from year to year.

The VA makes a random selection of three sample aids for each submitted stock model from the participating manufacturer's inventory. All aids are tested for the VA by the Automated Production Technology Division at NIST (the National Institute of Standards and Technology) and the Biocommunications Laboratory of the Catholic University of America, according to VA specified procedures.

The raw test data from NIST are statistically managed by the VA's National Hearing Aid Program staff from the Audiology and Speech Pathology Service, VA Medical Center, Washington, DC. An Index of Characteristics score—a measure of overall performance of a hearing aid model relative to other models—is computed for all regular hearing aid stock models. Performance on a number of subtests, including harmonic distortion, equivalent input noise level, index of effectiveness, uniformity of slope, and product uniformity contributes to the final score for each hearing aid model.

The VA negotiates contracts for hearing aid models that:

1. have higher Index of Characteristics scores than other models
2. meet specified electroacoustic criteria
3. have satisfactory design features

SUMMARY OF HEARING AID TEST PROGRAM FOR CONTRACT YEARS 1992–93

Manufacturer	Model	Type[1]
Audiotone, Inc. 4120 Olson Memorial Hwy. Golden Valley, MN 55422	A-61 *A-70 C410	OE OE OB
Beltone Electronics 4201 W. Victoria Chicago, IL 60646	Concerto *Prima Std. *Suprimo	OB OE OE
Electone, Inc. P.O. Box 910 Winter Park, FL 32790	AM240 HF	OE
GN Danavox, Inc. 5600 Rowland Road Minnetonka, MN 55343	*107-2PP 125PP AGC-I *133PP	OB OE OE
Maico Hearing Instruments, Inc. 7375 Bush Lake Road Minneapolis, MN 55435	*G117V *MC031V *MC033V	
Oticon, Inc. P.O. Box 6724 29 Schoolhouse Road Somerset, NJ 08875-6724	*E38P *E40 *E42P	OE OE OE
Philips Hearing Instruments 91 McKee Drive Mahwah, NJ 07430	P47H S46-0 *S1594	OE OE OB
Phonak, Inc. P.O. Box 3017 850 E. Diehl Road Naperville, IL 60566	*Super Front PP C2 Super Front PP SC	
Qualitone 4931 W. 35th Street Minneapolis, MN 55410	DED TSM *TSNE	OE OE EG

Category[2]	Gain[3]	SSPL[3]	Index of Characteristics[4]
Strong	52.0	135.0	84.2
Mild	36.0	118.0	100.3
Strg./Ex. Strg.	64.0	147.0	56.2
Strg./Ex. Strg.	62.0	143.0	94.2
Moderage	46.0	132.0	138.9
Moderate	42.0	126.0	128.5
High Pass	63.0	145.0	93.5
	48.0	133.0	
	37.0	125.0	113.0
Strg./Ex. Strg.	23.0	116.0	
High Pass			
Mild/Mod.			
Mild	32.0	117.0	130.5
Moderate	42.0	127.0	146.5
Moderate	41.0	125.0	148.5
Mod./Strg.	50.0	134.0	119.7
High Pass	19.0	110.0	
Moderate	43.0	129.0	122.9
High Pass	39.0	127.0	
Moderate	50.0	133.0	93.4
Strg./Ex. Strg.	61.0	145.0	48.6
Moderate	51.0	132.0	108.5
Moderate	48.0	128.0	90.2
High Pass	26.0	113.0	
Mild	38.0	121.0	88.0
Mild/Moderate	40.0	125.0	122.9

Manufacturer	Model	Type[1]
Rexton, Inc. 2415 Xenium Lane Plymouth, MN 55441	*Mini Primo PPI-G-C PP142 *Selectra PP-6	 OE OE OE
Siemens Hearing Instruments, Inc. 10 Constitution Avenue Piscataway, NJ 08854	408W-H 604PP	OE OE
Starkey Laboratories, Inc. 6700 Washington Avenue S. Eden Prairie, MN 55344	*AL PP-II *EuroStar VFC Star 42PP AI	
Telex Communications, Inc. 9600 Aldrich Avenue S. Minneapolis, MN 55420	338 MC *340 CLO *350 BC 366 *402 BC *402 C 402 MC	OE OE OE OE EG EG EG
Telstar, Inc. 4116 Cedar Avenue Minneapolis, MN 55407	700	OB
Unitron Industries, Inc. P.O. Box 5010 3555 Walnut Street Port Huron, MI 48061-5010	*UM60-PPA UM60-UH *US80-PPLA	OE OE OE

[1] **Type:** (EG) eyeglass; (OE) over-the-ear; (OB) on-the-body

[2] **Category:** Categories indicate specific types of instruments or are based on a specific Gain/SSPL range for regular models:

Mild (gain, 26–40 dB; SSPL, 106–121 dB)
Moderate (gain, 41–51 dB; SSPL, 122–133 dB)
Strong (gain, 52+ dB; SSPL, 134–142 dB)
Extra Strong (SSPL, 140+ dB)

[3] **Gain and SSPL (Saturation Sound Pressure Level):** Represent the mean figures for three samples of a model.

Category[2]	Gain[3]	SSPL[3]	Index of Characteristics[4]
Moderate	46.0	129.0	130.2
Strong	56.0	138.0	91.1
Moderate	50.0	133.0	107.7
High Pass	23.0	111.0	
Strong	54.0	136.0	74.5
Mod./Strg.	52.0	133.0	112.8
High Pass	35.0	127.0	
Strong	52.0	135.0	95.4
BICROS	47.0	128.0	
CROS	14.0	105.0	
BICROS	30.0	116.0	
Strong	53.0	136.0	57.4
BICROS	45.0	130.0	
CROS	25.0	114.0	
BICROS	45.0	130.0	
Strg./Ex. Strg.	60.0	142.0	52.4
Moderate	45.0	130.0	128.6
High Pass	23.0	120.0	
Mod./Strg.	49.0	135.0	139.6

[4] **Index of Characteristics:** A measure of the total performance of a stock hearing aid model relative to all other models submitted. The mean weighted scores of each model for the subtests of harmonic distortion, equivalent input noise level, index of effectiveness, uniformity of slope, and product uniformity are summed to provide the measure of total performance. *Note:* It is not computed for the CROS and High Pass categories, since some of the measurements needed to calculate the Index of Characteristics are not performed.

*Hearing aid models selected for Contract Year 1992–93 and those instruments scoring above the mean Index of Characteristics.

In the list on pages 236–39, hearing aids that score in the top 50 percent, together with those awarded a VA contract because they possess particular characteristics needed for special clinical problems, are marked with an asterisk (*). This is not to say that the remaining instruments are not of value. It simply means they did not perform as well on tests, and/or that they did not have characteristics judged to be as appropriate for the veteran population as others did. Additionally, the number of different manufacturers and models on contract is limited by administrative constraints in managing such a large program.

The VA does not test all hearing aids—only those submitted by manufacturers who want to participate in the VA program. Furthermore, manufacturers are limited to a specific number of models that they may submit, depending on VA requirements for each particular type. Some manufacturers do not participate at all in the VA's program, and others submit only one or two models for consideration. *The VA lists should not be used as an absolute buying guide. Aids not listed should not automatically be considered inferior devices.*

Primarily, the VA provides hearing aids only to veterans whose hearing disability is the result of military service. For further information, these veterans should contact their nearest VA facility. Other veterans and all nonveterans interested in hearing aids are advised to seek professional guidance in their local communities.

There is no "best" hearing aid for all individuals. Aids that test well for one person may not perform well for someone else. In addition, aids with certain special characteristics will not be appropriate for every type of hearing loss. It is important to note, therefore, that the hearing aid model with the highest Index of Characteristics score may not be the best one for you. The VA's general advice to a person with a hearing disability is to seek professional guidance in obtaining the aid best suited to the particular problem.

APPENDIX B

Consumer Reports Evaluation of Assistive Listening Devices

The Technical Division of *Consumer Reports* examined 26 devices from the hundreds of assistive listening devices (ALDs) on the market. In order to gain an overview of what was available, its engineers chose to evaluate several products within three groups of products. These three groups include devices that are related to:

- Telephone use
- Room listening (e.g., personal TV amplifier other than hearing aid)
- Alerting (e.g., vibrational/visual indication of a ringing doorbell)

In a few cases, more than one of a given type of product (from more than one manufacturer) was examined in order to do a limited comparison. Several hearing-impaired persons also examined the products on an informal basis and added their comments and experience to this report.

All products were purchased by mail order. The price paid is listed, but shipping costs are not included.

Most of the devices examined are helpful whether you use a hearing aid or not. Many people with mild to moderate hearing loss do not need a powerful hearing aid, only higher volume sound than others in the family. (Although hearing aids were used as an adjunct to tests, *Consumer Reports*' Technical Division did not examine hearing aids.) Some of the products work only if a hearing aid with a T-coil is available—the T-switch on hearing aids switches from acoustic pickup to the magnetic pickup that is required to use a hearing aid–compatible phone.

All of the evaluated devices functioned reasonably well. Elderly people, or those who are not able to operate modern electronic equipment, might be intimidated by some. Once set up, however, the devices are simple enough to use for most people.

AT&T and Plantronics Amplifiers

Both these amplifiers plug into the telephone between the telephone handset and the phone base. The *AT&T* unit uses a 9-volt battery to power the amplifier and the *Plantronics* unit has an AC adaptor that needs to be plugged into a 120-volt outlet.

While an ordinary phone handset produces about 75 decibels (dB) at the ear, these units allow sound pressure levels to be varied from about 75 to 95 dB. (An increase of 9 dB is generally perceived as "twice as loud.") A volume control unit on the small amplifier box (roughly 2 × 3 × 1½ inches) allows you to change volume. The box has a wire 8 to 10 inches long that must be plugged into the phone base; the phone's coiled handset wire can be plugged into the little box. Both of these devices worked on either the new electronic-type phone or the old-style (prior to breakup of AT&T) black desk phones. The *AT&T* Amplifier is about $29, the *Plantronics* unit is about $30.

Whistle Stop EA-K1

People using hearing aids without any T-coil sometimes experience an annoyingly loud whistle. This occurs because loud sound from the earpiece sometimes reaches the hearing aid transmitter, producing unwanted feedback. This simple device clips over a phone earpiece and helps prevent the sound from feeding back from the earpiece. Both rectangular and round-shaped *Whistle Stop* models are available to fit various phones. The unit costs about $12.

AT&T and Walker Amplified Handsets

Amplified telephone handsets are often very useful in noisy environments where someone with even slight hearing problems has difficulty hearing. The *ATT* and *Walker* amplified handsets replace the handset on old-style telephones. The handsets have a volume control and get their amplifier power from the phone line.

The *Walker* unit ($58) allows the sound level at the ear to be increased from normal to about 20 dB over a standard phone. The *AT&T* unit ($38) provided a range of plus or minus 10 dB relative to the standard. Neither of these handsets worked with modern electronic phones; most phones purchased in stores today are electronic and would not be compatible with these units.

Genesis K/G100 Amplified Handset

The *Genesis* amplified handset ($60) works on both modern electronic and on old-style phones. Amplification is variable from about 5 dB less to 25 dB more than standard. Steady loud sounds, such as a dial tone or room noise, are reduced in volume while intermittent voice peaks on the phone are amplified more. The *Genesis* model also boosts high frequencies to further help people with the common problem of high-frequency hearing loss. While some other amplified handsets will squeal if placed on a table, this unit automatically stops the squeal. This "smart" phone has features that are very desirable. The *Genesis* requires one AAA cell to power its amplifier.

AT&T Portable Amplifier

This strap-on amplifier boosts the volume coming from an ordinary telephone handset by 10 to 20 dB.

To use this amplifier, you slip its somewhat stiff rubber band around your phone's earpiece and turn a knob that serves as both On/Off switch and volume control. The amplifier is powered by an AAA-size battery.

The amplifier weighs about 2 ounces and measures about 2 inches square and ¾ of an inch thick. There are no wires to connect or unplug (as when installing an amplified handset or amplifier box) when using this portable device. It comes with a soft pouch so that you can carry it with you in your pocket or purse. This device costs about $25.

Cordless phones being used outdoors in noisy areas are more likely than corded phones to benefit from using this type of earpiece amplifier. Because the amplifier must be removed for the phone to fit in the cradle of a phone base, a cordless phone is less troublesome to use since the phone can be hung up by the push of a switch on the handset. The amplifier can be left on the handset all day—it has to be removed only at night when the cordless handset battery is being recharged.

Koss JCK/300 Cordless Headset

The *Koss* cordless headset is handy for the person who needs higher volume TV or stereo sound than required by others in the room. You plug a wireless infrared (IR) transmitter (supplied with headset) into the TV and then put the headset or earphones on and adjust the volume at the headset to suit yourself. The system transmits full stereo from stereo sources.

The transmitter, a flat 8 × 4 × 1½-inch box, is mounted on a slightly larger electronics box. The headset works fine up to about 20 feet away, but overhead fluorescent lights in the laboratory caused noise and prevented longer-range testing; the home living room is not likely to have this problem. (A range of 50 feet is possible but noise gets worse at greater range.) These units cannot be used outside in the sunlight.

Turning your head sometimes weakens the signal and introduces noise, but this is not a serious problem in most cases.

The headset has a volume control and requires a 9-volt battery. It weighs ¾ lb., but padding on top makes it comfortable for most people. Several people in a room can wear headphones and receive the same sound via the IR transmitter. The *Koss* unit has a price tag of $274.

Infrasound IR500 Cordless Headset

The *Infrasound* headset uses the same general IR technique as the *Koss* unit but the headset is lighter in weight (⅓ lb.) and lower in price ($110). It's also less bulky because it does not cover the ears as much as the *Koss* phones. (The *Koss* phones do help to keep out other sounds.) The transmitter is also more compact (about 8 × 3 × 3 inches) and looks more streamlined. This headset uses two small AAA cells to power the amplifier. Like the *Koss* transmitter, the *Infrasound* unit uses an AC adaptor to power the IR transmitter. While lower in cost, the *Infrasound* is monophonic, and sound is of lower quality than the *Koss*. The headset was judged not as comfortable as the *Koss*, but comfortable enough.

Williams Pocketalker PKT SYS B1

This device is relatively well known in the assistive hearing device field, and it has been found to be quite useful for both non–hearing aid and hearing aid users. (*AT&T* sells a *Pocketalker*—not tested—that looks exactly like the *Williams* device.) Similar to an old-fashioned "out-in-the-open" hearing aid, and small enough (about 2½ × 3½ × ¾ inches) to fit in a shirt pocket, the *Williams Pocketalker* has a microphone (covered with a windscreen to minimize wind noise) that protrudes ¾ inch or so to pick up room sounds. The unit sends the amplified sounds directly via wire to an earphone. The earphone that came with this unit hangs over the top of the ear (museums sometimes use this style) and does not fall out as easily as one that is pushed into the ear. A volume control on the top of the *Pocketalker* allows the user to conveniently adjust the listening sound level.

The *Pocketalker* ($134) comes with a cord 12 feet long so that the microphone can be placed across the room if desired—say, near a TV speaker. The person then attaches himself or herself to the wire running to the microphone. A belt-mountable carrying case comes with the unit.

Williams NKL001 Neckloop

When this wire (about a one-foot-long loop with an 18-inch wire and plug) is slipped under a shirt collar and plugged into the earphone jack of the *Pocketalker* (or other audio source), it creates a magnetic field that a hearing aid user can use when the aid is left in the "T" mode. (Some hearing aids do not have a T-coil and cannot make use of the neckloop or of hearing aid–compatible telephones' magnetic fields.) An *Electone* Model AM92PP behind-the-ear hearing aid was used with a T-coil in the tests. The neckloop can be used with other audio sources such as tape recorders and television sets and not just with the *Pocketalker*. An 8-to-16-ohm audio output through a small-style jack is the recommended connection to the *Neckloop*, which is priced at $37.

Williams Personal FM

This system allows the user to place the microphone near a sound source, such as a TV, and transmit the sound via FM radio waves across the room. In effect, it is much like the IR system described earlier. The receiver and transmitter are of the same size as the *Pocketalker*. Both the transmitter and the receiver came with belt-mountable carrying cases; two people could have a one-way radio link with this system, which has an unobstructed range of over 200 feet. Being radio-operated, the receiver (depending on wall construction) can often be used in a different room than the transmitter. The earphone supplied is a foam-cushioned type that pushes into the ear. (*Williams* offers several earphone options.) The receiver is compatible with the *Williams Neckloop* so that a hearing aid in the "T" position can be used to hear the desired sound without interference by surrounding room noise. At times, in our tests, other VHF (very high frequency) radio conversations were picked up on this system when it was used outside of the building, but interference is not a serious problem in normal use. If more than one of these systems is to be used in the same building, *Williams* offers four different VHF frequencies to prevent systems from interfering with each other. The *Williams* Personal FM costs about $446.

Rastronics Mini1000 Teleloop System

Audio induction loops have long been used in classrooms, museums, and other public places. This personal induction loop device ($185) is gaining popularity in the home. Up to two microphones or other audio inputs (such as TV) can be connected to the *Rastronics* transmitter (an 8 × 4½ × 2-inch box). By placing a long piece of wire under a rug or under a molding near the ceiling and attaching the wire to the *Rastronics* transmitter, the sound fed to the transmitter can be picked up by a hearing aid equipped with a T-coil almost any place in the room. This unit comes with 100 feet of wire for the loop. In walking around the test room with a T-coil-equipped hearing aid, a few dead spots were found, but most locations in the room allowed the examiners to clearly pick up the sound fed to the transmitter.

Quest Silent Page Basic System

The *Quest* system consists of a wrist receiver on an expansion band—the device itself resembles a big wristwatch. The wrist receiver vibrates to notify the person that an alert condition exists. The wrist receiver has an On/Off switch that is unmarked as to which position is Off. It also has a reset switch to stop the vibrator, and five tiny lights on the wrist receiver. The top light is labeled "T" to indicate that the telephone is ringing. The other four lights are numbered; the alert condition indicated by these lights depends upon how the alerting transmitters are set. The user could write something next to the numbers on the wrist receiver to identify the specific alert indicated by each light.

The basic system used in the evaluation came with two alerting transmitters, each of which operates with 9-volt batteries. The transmitters (about 4½ × 3¼ × 1½ inches) send radio signals to the wrist receiver, causing it to vibrate. Each detects acoustic sounds via an internal microphone. For example, the transmitter can be placed next to a telephone or doorbell, where the loud ring will trigger operation. Three switch settings on the transmitter allow you to send an alarm if the sound is of long, medium, or of short duration; almost any short-term noise or sound triggers the device in the short-term position. Inside the transmitter are tiny DIP switches that allow you to change the vibration pattern of the wrist receiver so that the wearer can identify the noise source by feel. The transmitter has a range of about 70 feet across an unobstructed line of sight. The system is priced at $440.

Quest MCII Manual Paging Device

This unit ($200) is essentially like the sound-actuated transmitter described above but is actuated by pushing a button on the top of the box instead of by a microphone picking up loud sounds. Thus you can page the person wearing the wrist receiver.

Quest SP II Basic Receiver

Another set of *Quest* units has a wrist receiver that does not have lights to identify the sound source; the wearer must remember the vibration pattern if there is more than one transmitter to alert him or her to different conditions. Except for the lack of lights, this receiver looks exactly like the unit with lights. Both use a special 7-volt mercury battery that is available through *Radio Shack* stores for $5.89. *Note:* The battery must have part of the label shaved off before it will fit into the battery compartment. This battery problem could be rather inconvenient, but a "shaved" battery is available directly from *Quest* for $6.50 plus shipping.

As described, the transmitters must be programmed to actuate the wrist receiver. It may be difficult for some people to master this task. Just getting the cover off of the transmitter to replace the 9-volt battery is likely to be a problem for some. The *Quest* sells for about $240.

Silent Call 1001 System Receiver

This alerting device was designed to be worn clipped to a belt. When the unit receives a radio signal from a transmitter, it vibrates. (Several transmitters, called pagers by *Silent Call*, are described below.) The vibration is strong enough to be detected by virtually anyone, despite intervening clothing, and the buzz of the vibrator is clearly audible to persons with normal hearing. The top of the belt-mounted receiver has four lights that tell which of four transmitters is sending the alert signal. The lights are labeled Phone, Door, Sound, and Fire. Icon-type pictures (flame, etc.) next to the lights caption the alerting light. A clearly labeled On/Off switch is also located on the top of this somewhat bulky (5 × 3 × 1¼-inch) box. A clear range between transmitter and receiver of over 80 feet was realized. A 9-volt battery powers this unit, which costs about $120.

Silent Call 1004 Manual Pager

This manual pager ($50) transmits a signal that causes the *Silent Call 1001* receiver to intermittently vibrate on and off while the paging button is depressed. It does not cause a light to go on at the receiver. The unit is 4½ × 2¼ × 1 inches, uses a 9-volt battery, and comes with a belt clip.

Silent Call 1003 Doorbell Pager

This unit is the same size as the manual pager, but it has wires that connect it to the doorbell. A recessed push button used on this unit is like one on the manual pager, but here it functions as a test button to show that the battery is OK; a light goes on when its transmitter is actuated by the doorbell or the test button. This unit sells for about $50.

Silent Call 1002 Telephone Pager

Similar to the bell pager, this unit ($50) plugs into the telephone line in the same manner as a phone. When the phone rings or the test button is pushed on this unit, the belt-mounted receiver vibrates, and the telephone lights on the receiver and pager glow.

Sonic Alert WA300 Light Blinker

For people who can't be awakened by an acoustic alarm, this device ($45) turns a lamp on and off intermittently. The WA300 plugs into a 120-volt outlet, and a lamp (200-watt maximum incandescent) is plugged into it. An alarm clock (or any loud device) can be placed on top of or next to the unit, and the sound causes the lamp to start blinking. A single ring will cause several blinks; the number of blinks depends upon the duration of the ring.

Sonic Alert TR55 Phone Ring Pager

This unit plugs into a 120-volt outlet and a separate wire plugs into the phone line. When the phone rings, a lamp plugged into this signaler blinks intermittently. When the *TR55* was unplugged from a 120-volt wall socket, the plastic back of the device fell off because of weak construction. The unit, priced at $46, can handle an incandescent lamp of up to 300 watts.

Gentex 710 LS Strobe Light Smoke Detector

The severely hearing-impaired person may not hear an ordinary home smoke detector alarm. This 120-volt (plug-in, power-line-operated) smoke detector has a very bright blinking strobe light and an extra loud (120 dB) audible alarm. The strobe light is about as bright as a camera flash unit. Strobe lights are often used with other systems to alert hearing-impaired people who may not notice an ordinary incandescent blinker. The *Gentex* sells for about $136.

Rexton Pillow Vibrator

This battery-operated (one C cell) alarm clock comes with a vibrator designed to be put under a pillow. The vibrator is shaped like a flying saucer (3¾-inch dia. × ¾-inch thick at middle) and is attached to a 6-foot wire that plugs into the back of the clock. It is not at all uncomfortable under a pillow, and the vibration is sufficient to awaken the average person. When the alarm goes off, the user only has to tap the top of the clock to shut the alarm off. (When the pillow vibrator is plugged in, the clock alarm does not sound.) Without the vibrator, an alarm ring of 86 dB (adequate for those with fair-to-good hearing) emanates from the clock. The quartz-controlled clock, 3 inches in diameter with a sweep second hand, keeps good time. The unit is priced at $55.

Hal-Hen Shake & Wake Bed Vibrator

This wake-up device, designed to be bolted or screwed to a bed headboard or frame, consists of a deliberately out-of-balance 120-volt AC motor. A *Hal-Hen* clock timer (described below) must be bought separately to turn on the vibrator. When the vibrator is merely slipped between a mattress and box spring at one corner, it shakes the bed vigorously; however, this placement is a temporary setup and may cause the mattress to stick up in an awkward manner. No instructions are included. The unit sells for about $45. Includes a rugged 9-foot-long power cord with an On/Off power switch that is 3 feet from the motor.

Hal-Hen Timer (for above vibrator)

Hal-Hen sells this timer ($46) for the deaf and hard-of-hearing and recommends it for use with the above *Hal-Hen* vibrator. The clock timer has a snooze button and a battery tester for its backup 9-volt battery. If power is cut off, the battery keeps the clock from losing time, but then the digital time display does not work. The timer can turn on a lamp, TV, or some other wake-up device. The AC outlet on the back of the timer is rated at 1,195 watts, which is enough for the bed vibrator or a bright strobe lamp. The 1-inch-high numerals on the digital time readout should be helpful to the visually impaired.

Recommendations

In general, it is desirable to consult an otolaryngologist or audiologist for recommendations on appropriate devices.

Readers should be aware that there are many devices on the market similar to the devices examined, and it is quite possible that many of these similar devices combine good quality and low prices. Send for catalogs or visit a store, if one is available, where you can directly examine and possibly test the various units. (See list of names and addresses of suppliers at the end of this appendix.)

Those who cannot hear well enough to use a telephone may wish to consider acquiring a TDD or TT (telecommunications device for the deaf). Under the Americans with Disabilities Act (ADA), TDDs will soon be required in some public places. (Sometimes the name TTY is used, because old-fashioned, large teletypewriters—traditionally abbreviated TTY—have been used for this purpose.) TDDs have keyboards to type messages as well as visual displays to show incoming messages and outgoing messages. Some can store entire telephone-typed conversations. While only 20 characters at a time can be shown typically, many TDDs can be attached to a printer to put the conversation on paper. A device can be used to alert a TDD user that there is an incoming call.

Other choices available to the hearing-impaired include personal FAX machines, closed-captioned TV boxes, beepers that vibrate and display messages, and even hearing-ear dogs (see page 226).

While most of the products examined do what they were designed to do, these devices are sometimes less attractive and are somewhat bulkier than good-quality consumer electronic products. If you search for a general consumer device that can do the same job, you might find a better design or price. Sometimes a consumer product can be modified for the hearing-impaired.

For example, the *Koss* infrared (IR) system is a general consumer product that is available in discount stores because it is used by many stereo enthusiasts to listen to music privately, without bothering other people in the same room. Some lower-cost monaural IR devices are also on the general market.

AT&T phone stores handle a few devices for the hearing-impaired, but some of their advertised products must be ordered by mail from their National Special Needs Center. *Radio Shack* stores also sell some useful devices for the hearing-impaired, but not all catalog items are stocked in all stores. A few mail-order firms specializing in the ALD field have walk-in stores where the items can be observed and explained by salespeople who are very familiar with the products.

Learning to use the devices is important, too. For instance, many people do not know how to use their hearing aid with a hearing aid–compatible telephone. There is only one small spot on the earpiece where the hearing aid can pick up a strong signal, so one simply has to move the earpiece a little to find it. All of the devices evaluated here need to be thoroughly studied by the user and friends or family to determine their suitability for any given individual, and the hearing-impaired person then may need help in operating them to their maximum potential.

Sources of Assistive Listening Devices

Note: "A" means alerting devices; "T" means telephone devices; "G" means general devices; and "Y" means TT or TDD devices are available.

Accessible Communications Products Center — A, T, G, Y
5 Wood Hollow Road, Rm. 1119
Parsippany, NJ 07054
(800) 233-1222

Audex — G
713 N. Fourth Street
Longview, TX 75601
(903) 753-7058

Audio Enhancement — G
8 Winfield Pointe Lane
St. Louis, MO 63141
(314) 567-6141

Audiophone Hearing Instruments — A, G, T
709 Pere Marquette Bldg.
150 Barone Street
New Orleans, LA 70112
(504) 524-8124

Auditory Instruments — G
4699 Auvergne #17
Lisle, IL 60532
(708) 963-0505

Comtek, Inc. 357 W. 2700 S. Salt Lake City, UT 84115 (801) 466-3463	G
Dahlberg, Inc. 4101 Dahlberg Drive Golden Valley, MN 55422 (612) 520-9705	G
Earmark 1125 Dixwell Avenue Hamden, CT 06514 (203) 777-2130	G
Eckstein Brothers, Inc. 4807 W. 118th Place Hawthorne, CA 90250 (213) 772-6113	G
Everett Assistive Resources Co. P.O. Box 3353 Everett, WA 98203 (800) 669-7371	T
Exceptional Hearing Services, Inc. 515 Northgate Drive San Rafael, CA 94903 (415) 499-7766	A, G
Guinta Associates, Inc. 37 Terhune Avenue Lodi, NJ 07644 (201) 773-8284	A, G, T, Y
Hal-Hen 35-53 24th Street Long Island City, NY 11106 (800) 242-5436	A, G, T, Y

HARC Mercantile Ltd. 3130 Portage Street P.O. Box 3055 Kalamazoo, MI 49003 (616) 381-0177	A, G, T, Y
Hear You Are, Inc. 4 Musconetcong Avenue Stanhope, NJ 07874 (201) 347-7662	A, G, T, Y
Instrumentation Associates Trolley Crossing Office Park 8116 Cazenovia Road Manlius, NY 13104 (315) 682-2600	A, G, T
J. W. Manny, Inc. 48 E. 43rd Street New York, NY 10017 (212) 682-7956	G
Med-Tec, Inc. 3 Orchard Avenue Watkins Glen, NY 14891 (800) 400-5402	A, G, T, Y
Metavox, Inc. 8375 Leesburg Pike, Ste. 421 Vienna, VA 22182 (703) 698-0802	G
National Hearing Aid Distributors, Inc. 145 Tremont Street Boston, MA 02111 (617) 426-9845	A, G, T, Y
Nationwide Flashing Signal Systems 8120 Fenton Street Silver Spring, MD 20910 (301) 589-6671	A, G, T, Y

Oticon, Inc. G
29 Schoolhouse Road
Somerset, NJ 08873
(908) 560-1220

Parente Associates, Inc. G
P.O. Box 113
Cheshire, CT 06410
(203) 272-5123

Phonak, Inc. G
850 E. Diehl Road
P.O. Box 3017
Naperville, IL 60566
(800) 777-7333

Radio Shack A, G, T
1500 One Tandy Center
Fort Worth, TX 76102
(817) 390-3011

R&M Communications Products A, G, T, Y
9203 W. Bluemound Road
Wauwatosa, WI 53226
(414) 475-7770

Rexton, Inc. A
2415 Xenium Lane
Plymouth, MN 55441
(800) 876-1141

Rion Co., Ltd. G
P.O. Box 18007
West St. Paul, MN 55118
(612) 457-2177

Sennheiser Electronic Corp. G
6 Vista Drive
P.O. Box 987
Old Lyme, CT 06371
(203) 434-9190

Sound Associates, Inc. 424 W. 45th Street New York, NY 10036 (212) 757-5679	G
Telex Communications, Inc. 3510 Mainway P.O. Box 1488, Sta. B Burlington, Ontario CANADA L7R 4L9 (416) 335-3744	G
Ultratec, Inc. 450 Science Drive Madison, WI 53711 (608) 238-5400	Y
Unitron Industries, Inc. 3555 Walnut Street P.O. Box 5010 Port Huron, MI 48061 (313) 982-0166	G
Jay L. Warren, Inc. P.O. Box 25413 Chicago, IL 60625 (312) 275-1525	G
Weitbrecht Communications, Inc. 2656 29th Street, Ste. 205 Santa Monica, CA 90405 (800) 233-9130	A, G, T, Y
Williams Sound Corp. 10399 W. 70th Street Eden Prairie, MN 55344 (800) 843-3544	G, T
Wilner-Greene Associates 449 Forest Avenue Plaza Portland, ME 04101 (800) 634-4327	A, G, T, Y

APPENDIX C

Sources of Additional Information

Alexander Graham Bell Association for the Deaf, Inc.
3417 Volta Place N.W.
Washington, DC 20007
(202) 337-5220

Provides information on hearing loss in children and adults and works to promote better understanding of hearing loss by the public. Promotes early detection of hearing loss in infants. Offers information on oral communication and provides information on where speech-reading lessons are available nationwide.

American Academy of Audiology
P.O. Box 3676
Washington, DC 20007
(202) 687-6997
(800) 222-2336

This professional organization establishes educational and professional guidelines and requirements for audiologists. Provides names of qualified audiologists to consumers by geographic region upon request.

American Academy of Otolaryngology—Head and Neck Surgery
One Prince Street
Alexandria, VA 22314
(703) 836-4444

Offers information about medicine relating to otolaryngology or head and neck surgery. Provides pamphlets discussing medical problems of the ear and referrals to physicians.

American Speech-Language-Hearing Association
10801 Rockville Pike
Rockville, MD 20852
(301) 897-5700
(800) 638-8255 (Consumer Helpline)

This professional organization for speech-language pathologists and audiologists provides a variety of informational materials to consumers on speech, language, and hearing problems.

American Tinnitus Association
P.O. Box 5
Portland, OR 97207
(503) 248-9985

Provides information about tinnitus and support groups around the country. Promotes public information about tinnitus.

Better Hearing Institute
5021-B Backlick Road
Annandale, VA 22003
(703) 642-0580
(800) EAR-WELL

Provides information on hearing loss, types of available help, and sources of assistance.

The EAR Foundation
2000 Church Street
Box 111
Nashville, TN 37236
(615) 329-7809
(800) 545-HEAR

Offers public and professional educational programs and support services related to hearing and balance problems. Administers the Ménière's Network, a national network of support groups for people with Ménière's disease.

Hearing Education and Awareness for Rockers—H.E.A.R.
P.O. Box 460847
San Francisco, CA 94146
(415) 773-9590

Offers educational programs on how repeated exposure to loud noise endangers hearing and causes hearing loss. H.E.A.R. has a 24-hour hot line that provides information on hearing loss, protection of hearing, and how to get help.

HEAR NOW
4001 S. Magnolia Way
Denver, CO 80237
(303) 758-4919
(800) 648-HEAR

Raises funds to provide hearing aids and cochlear implants to adults and children who have a hearing loss but lack the financial means to buy such devices on their own.

International Hearing Society
20361 Middlebelt Road
Livonia, MI 48152
(313) 478-2610
(800) 521-5247

This professional association of hearing aid dispensers provides consumer information through its toll-free Hearing Aid Helpline.

John Tracy Clinic
806 W. Adams Boulevard
Los Angeles, CA 90007
(213) 748-5481
(800) 522-4582

Offers correspondence courses free of charge to parents whose preschool children are deaf or hard-of-hearing.

National Information Center on Deafness
Gallaudet University
800 Florida Avenue N.E.
Washington, DC 20002
(202) 651-5051

The NICD collects, develops, and disseminates information about all aspects of hearing loss as well as services available to deaf and hard-of-hearing people nationwide. NICD offers a complete list of national nonprofit organizations of interest to deaf or hard-of-hearing people. NICD also provides information about Gallaudet University, a liberal arts university for deaf students.

National Technical Institute for the Deaf
Rochester Institute of Technology
One Lomb Memorial Drive
P.O. Box 9887
Rochester, NY 14623
(716) 475-6400

Provides postsecondary education in technological studies for deaf and hard-of-hearing students.

Rehabilitation Services Administration
Communications Impairment Section
605 G Street N.W., Suite 1021
Washington, DC 20001
(202) 727-0981

Provides rehabilitation services for deaf and hard-of-hearing people as well as those with speech or language impairments. This agency provides technical assistance to state rehabilitation agencies, other agencies, and to individuals.

Self-Help for Hard-of-Hearing People (SHHH)
7800 Wisconsin Avenue
Bethesda, MD 20814
(301) 657-2248

This self-help and support organization provides information, education, referral, and advisory services to the hearing-impaired and to interested people with normal hearing. Promotes public awareness of hearing loss, assistive listening devices, and alternative communciation skills.

Tele-Consumer Hotline
1910 K Street N.W., Suite 610
Washington, DC 20006
(202) 223-4371
(800) 332-1124

This consumer information service provides telephone assistance and publications. Those interested may inquire about special telephone equipment, telephone selection, troubleshooting information, and consumer advice on avoiding fraud.

Vestibular Disorders Association
P.O. Box 4467
Portland, OR 97208-4467
(503) 229-7705

Provides information and support for people with vestibular disorders, and develops public and professional awareness of the issues associated with these disorders.

REFERENCES

Ackerman, D. A *Natural History of the Senses.* New York: Random House, 1990.

Alexander, L. "Deaf Students Education Services: Policy Guidance." *Federal Register* 57, no. 211 (October 30, 1992): 49274–49276.

American Academy of Audiology. Position Statement. "Graduate Education." *Audiology Today* 2, no. 5 (September–October 1990): 10.

American Academy of Otolaryngology—Head and Neck Surgery. *Assistive Communication Devices.* 1989.

American Academy of Otolaryngology—Head and Neck Surgery. *Cochlear Implant: A Device to Help the Deaf Hear.* 1990.

American Academy of Otolaryngology—Head and Neck Surgery. *Doctor, What Causes the Noise in My Ears?* 1989.

American Academy of Otolaryngology—Head and Neck Surgery. *Ears, Altitude and Airplane Travel.* 1990.

American Academy of Otolaryngology—Head and Neck Surgery. *Noise, Ears and Hearing Protection.* 1990.

American Speech-Language-Hearing Association. "Assistive Devices and Listening Systems." *Let's Talk,* no. 37.

American Speech-Language-Hearing Association. "Communication with People with Hearing Impairment." *Let's Talk,* no. 34.

American Speech-Language-Hearing Association. *Fortune 500s Survey.* 1989.

American Speech-Language-Hearing Association. "Mail Order Hearing Aids." *Let's Talk,* no. 17.

American Speech-Language-Hearing Association. *Special Devices for People with Hearing Loss.* 1992.

"And What About Hearing Benefits?" *Business & Health,* August 1990.

Balkany, T. "A Brief Perspective on Cochlear Implants." *The New England Journal of Medicine* 328, no. 4 (January 28, 1993): 281–282.

Baloh, R. W. "Diagnosis and Treatment of the Dizzy Patient." *New Horizons in Otolaryngology/Head and Neck Surgery* 3, no. 2 (August 1984).

Baloh, R. W., and J. M. R. Furman. "Modern Vestibular Function Testing." *The Western Journal of Medicine* 150, no. 1 (January 1989): 59–67.

Barnett, R. "Ginger: Getting to the Root of Motion Sickness." *Travel & Leisure*, September 1987.

Beaulac, D. A., J. L. Pehringer, and L. F. Shough. "Assistive Listening Devices: Available Options." *Seminars in Hearing* 10, no. 1 (February 1989): 11–30.

Beck, L. B., and G. C. Nance. "Hearing Aids, Assistive Listening Devices, and Telephones: Issues to Consider." *Seminars in Hearing* 10, no. 1 (February 1989): 78–89.

Bennett, W. I. "Hearing Loss—Boom and Doom." *Harvard Medical School Health Letter* 16, no. 2 (December 1990): 1–4.

Berger, E. H. "Selection and Use of Hearing Protectors." *Seminars in Hearing* 9, no. 4 (November 1988): 309–323.

Berger, K. W. *The Hearing Aid: Its Operation and Development*. 3rd ed. Livonia, Michigan: National Hearing Aid Society, 1984.

"Better Communication Between Hard of Hearing and Hearing People." *SHHH Journal*, March/April 1989.

Brandt, T., and R. B. Daroff. "Physical Therapy for Benign Paroxysmal Positional Vertigo." *Arch Otolaryngol* 106 (August 1980): 484–485.

Browne, M. W. "Noise Experts Agree: America Is Land of Battered Eardrums." *The New York Times*, May 14, 1992.

Clark, W. W. "Hearing: The Effects of Noise." *Otolaryngology—Head and Neck Surgery* 106, no. 6 (June 1992): 669–676.

Clark, W. W. "Noise Exposure from Leisure Activities: A Review." *Journal of the Acoustical Society of America* 90, no. 1 (July 1991): 175–181.

"Cochlear Implants Can Help Deaf Children Comprehend Speech." *Family Practice News* 22, no. 2 (January 15, 1992): 8.

Cody, D. T. R. *Your Child's Ears, Nose, and Throat*. New York: Macmillan, 1974.

Combs, A. *Hearing Loss Help*. Santa Maria, California: Alpenglow, 1988.

Commission on Education of the Deaf. A Report to the President and Congress of the United States. *Toward Equality: Education of the Deaf*. Washington, DC: Superintendent of Documents, U.S. Government Printing Office, 1988.

Compton, C. L., L. DiPietro, and L. VanMiddlesworth. *The New Hearing Aids and You*. Washington, DC: National Information Center on Deafness, 1992.

Compton, C. L., L. VanMiddlesworth, and L. DiPietro. *All About the New Generation of Hearing Aids*. Washington, DC: National Information Center on Deafness, 1992.

Cornacchia, H. J., and S. Barrett. *Consumer Health*. St. Louis: Times Mirror/Mosby, 1989.

Crammatte, A. B. *Questions and Answers . . . About Employment of Deaf People*. Washington, DC: National Information Center on Deafness, 1991.

Davis, Hallowell, and S. Richard Silverman. *Hearing and Deafness*. 4th ed. New York: Holt, Rinehart and Winston, 1978.

"Decibel Overload." *Consumer Reports* 56, no. 9 (October 1991): 660.

DeWitt, K. "Making Pay Phones Friendly to the Deaf." *The New York Times*, December 12, 1990.

DiPietro, L., P. Williams, and H. Kaplan. *Alerting and Communication Devices for Hearing-Impaired People: What's Available Now*. Washington, DC: National Information Center on Deafness/American Speech-Language-Hearing Association, 1987.

Ezzell, C. "Hearing Gene." *Science News* 141 (May 2, 1992): 296–297.

Fay, T. H., ed. *Noise and Health*. New York: The New York Academy of Medicine, 1991.

Federal Trade Commission. "Hearing Aids." *Facts for Consumers*, May 1991.

"Financial Help for Hearing Aids." *SHHH Journal*, May /June 1991.

Flodin, K. "Now Hear This." *American Health* 11, no. 1 (January/February 1992): 58–62.

Freeland, A. P. *Deafness: The Facts*. New York: Oxford University Press, 1989.

Gasaway, D. C. "Hearing Protection Guide Directs Users to Manufacturers/Devices by Category." *Occupational Health and Safety*, May 1988.

Gasaway, D. C. "Noise-Induced Hearing Loss." In *Handbook of Occupational Medicine*. Edited by R. J. McCunney. Boston: Little, Brown, 1988.

Green, J. D., Jr., D. J. Blum, and S. G. Harner. "Longitudinal Follow-up of Patients with Ménière's Disease." *Otolaryngology—Head and Neck Surgery* 104, no. 6 (June 1991): 783–788.

Grundfast, K., and C. J. Carney. *Ear Infections in Your Child*. New York: Warner, 1987.

Gulya, A. J. "Neuroanatomy and Physiology of the Vestibular System Relevant to Dysequilibrium in the Elderly." *Ear, Nose, and Throat Journal* 68 (December 1989): 915–924.

Himber, C. *How to Survive Hearing Loss*. Washington, DC: Gallaudet, 1989.

Horak, F. B., C. Jones-Rycewicz, F. O. Black, and A. Shumway-Cook. "Effects of Vestibular Rehabilitation on Dizziness and Balance." *Otolaryngology—Head and Neck Surgery* 106, no. 2 (February 1992): 175–180.

"How to Buy a Hearing Aid." *Consumer Reports* 57, no. 11 (November 1992): 716–721.

International Hearing Society. *The World of Sound. Facts About Hearing and Hearing Aids*. Livonia, MI: 1992.

Jaret, P. "The Rock & Roll Syndrome." *In Health* 4, no. 4 (July/August 1990): 50–57.

Joint Committee on Infant Hearing. "1990 Position Statement." *American Academy of Otolaryngology—Head and Neck Surgery Bulletin*, March 1991, 15–18.

Kirkwood, D. "Hearing Loss Emerges as a High-Profile Healthcare Issue." *The Hearing Journal* 44, no. 7 (July 1991): 9–17.

Konrad, H. R., D. Tomlinson, C. W. Stockwell, M. Norre, F. B. Horak, N. T. Shepard, and S. J. Herdman. "Rehabilitation Therapy for Patients with Disequilibrium and Balance Disorders." *Otolaryngology—Head and Neck Surgery* 107, no. 1 (July 1992): 105–108.

Kosovich, G. "Getting Help with a Job." *SHHH Journal*, July/August 1990.

Lanpher, K., and K. Keller. "Turn Down That Noise." *Redbook*, April 1991.

Leary, W. E. "Risk of Hearing Loss Is Growing." *The New York Times*, January 25, 1990.

Leary, W. E. "U.S. Panel Backs Testing All Babies to Uncover Hearing Losses Early." *The New York Times*, March 19, 1993.

Leavitt, R. J. "Considerations for Use of Rehabilitation Technology by the Hearing-Impaired Person." *Seminars in Hearing* 10, no. 1 (February 1989): 1–10.

Lipman, M. M. "Hearing Loss: Don't Suffer in Silence." *Consumer Reports Health Letter* 3, no. 7 (July 1991): 54–55.

Loewenthal, T. *Assessment of Hearing. An Introduction to the Art.* In-service training materials for medical students and residents at The Children's Hospital, Boston, 1978.

Lucente, F. E., and S. M. Sobol, eds. *Essentials of Otolaryngology.* 2nd ed. New York: Raven Press, 1988.

Luterman, D. *Counseling Parents of Hearing-Impaired Children.* Boston: Little, Brown, 1979.

Luterman, D. M., and M. Ross. *When Your Child Is Deaf.* Parkton, Maryland: York, 1991.

Marmon, L. "Now Hear This." *Washington Post Health*, August 8, 1989.

Massachusetts Eye and Ear Infirmary. *Facts About Cochlear Implants.* Boston, 1984.

"Ménière's Disease: An Earful." *Harvard Medical School Health Letter* 13, no. 4 (February 1988): 1–2.

Ménière's Network. *An Introduction to Ménière's Disease*. Nashville, 1989.

Modeland, V. "When Bells Are Ringing (but There Aren't Any Bells). *FDA Consumer*, April 1989.

Moora, C. "Medicare Fees." *Audiology Today* 4, no. 3 (May/June 1992): 16–20.

Myerson, A. R. "Companies Prepare for New Law on Disabled." *The New York Times*, July 25, 1992.

Nadol, J. B. Jr., and H. F. Schuknecht. "The Pathology of Peripheral Vestibular Disorders in the Elderly." *Ear, Nose, and Throat Journal* 68 (December 1989): 930–934.

National Information Center on Deafness. *Assistive Devices Demonstration Centers*. Washington, DC, 1992.

National Information Center on Deafness. *Directory of National Organizations of and for Deaf and Hard of Hearing People*. Washington, DC, 1992.

National Information Center on Deafness. *Educating the Deaf and Hard of Hearing Child: A Legal Perspective*. Washington, DC, October 1992.

National Information Center on Deafness. *Hearing Aids and Other Assistive Devices: Where to Get Assistance*. Washington, DC, 1989.

National Information Center on Deafness. *Mainstreaming Deaf and Hard of Hearing Students: Questions & Answers*. Washington, DC, 1991.

National Institutes of Health Consensus Development Conference on Noise and Hearing Loss. *NIH Consensus Statement on Noise and Hearing Loss* 8, no. 1 (January 22–24, 1990).

National Institutes of Health. *Program and Abstracts*. NIH Consensus Development Conference on Noise and Hearing Loss. Bethesda, MD: January 22–24, 1990.

Newby, H. A., and G. A. Popelka. *Audiology*. 5th ed. Englewood Cliffs, NJ: Prentice-Hall, 1985.

Nicolosi, L., E. Harryman, and J. Kresheck. *Terminology of Communication Disorders*. Baltimore: Williams & Wilkins, 1989.

Noble, B. P. "When Businesses Need Not Fret" and "The Phony Disability Experts." *The New York Times*, June 7, 1992.

Noha, N. "Assistive Technology." *SHHH Journal*, July/August 1992.

Odkvist, L. M., C. Moller, and K. Thuomas. "Otoneurologic Disturbances Caused by Solvent Pollution." *Otolaryngology—Head and Neck Surgery* 106, no. 6 (June 1992): 687–692.

Palmer, J. M., and P. A. Yantis. *Survey of Communication Disorders*. Baltimore: Williams & Wilkins, 1990.

Resen, S. V., and C. Hausman. *Coping with Hearing Loss*. New York: Dembner, 1985.

Rochester Institute of Technology. National Technical Institute for the Deaf, National Center on Employment of the Deaf. *Tips for Communicating with Deaf Employees*. Rochester, NY, 1987.

Rochester Institute of Technology. National Technical Institute for the Deaf, National Center on Employment of the Deaf. *Working Side by Side: Deaf and Hearing Colleagues*. Rochester, NY, 1992.

Rosenthal, R. *The Hearing Loss Handbook*. New York: Schocken Books, 1978.

Ruben, B. "On Deaf Ears." *Environmental Action*, March/April 1991.

Rybak, L. P. "Hearing: The Effects of Chemicals." *Otolaryngology—Head and Neck Surgery* 106, no. 6 (June 1992): 677–686.

Samuels, M. A. "Doctor, I'm Dizzy." *Brigham and Women's Hospital Medical Update* 2, no. 2 (September 1989).

Samuels, M. A. "Vertigo." *Harvard Medical School Health Letter* 15, no. 5 (March 1990): 6–8.

Sataloff, J. *Hearing Loss*. Philadelphia: J. B. Lippincott, 1966.

Schein, J. D. "Hearing-Impaired People in the Workplace." *SHHH Journal*, May/June 1987.

Schmeck, H. M., Jr. "Expert Panel Affirms Success of Ear Implants for the Profoundly Deaf." *The New York Times*, May 5, 1988.

Schwartz, S., ed. *Choices in Deafness*. Kensington, Maryland: Woodbine House, 1987.

Shimon, D. A. *Coping with Hearing Loss and Hearing Aids*. San Diego: Singular, 1992.

Shupert, C. L. *Labyrinthitis and Neuronitis: Infections of the Inner Ear*. Portland, OR: Vestibular Disorders Association, 1991.

Strome, M., J. Kelly, and M. Fried. *Manual of Otolaryngology*. Boston: Little, Brown, 1992.

Strome, M., and D. Vernick. "Hearing Loss and Hearing Aids." *Harvard Medical School Health Letter*, April 1989, 5–8.

"Swimmer's Ear." *Berkeley Wellness Letter* 7, issue 11 (August 1991): 6.

Technology Assessment Program and the National Center for Law and the Deaf, Gallaudet University, and the Bureau of Economic Research, Rutgers University. *Financing the Purchase of Devices for Deaf and Severely Hard of Hearing People: A Directory of Sources*. Washington, DC: Gallaudet Research Institute Monograph Series B, no. 3, 1989.

Thomsen, J. "Defining Valid Approaches to Therapy for Ménière's Disease." *Ear, Nose and Throat Journal* 65 (September 1986): 396–402.

"Tinnitus: When Your Ears Ring and Ring." *Berkeley Wellness Letter* 6, issue 6 (March 1990): 7.

University of Medicine and Dentistry of New Jersey—Robert Wood Johnson Medical School. *Health and Safety in Small Industry*. Chelsea, Michigan: Lewis, 1989.

U.S. Department of Justice. Civil Rights Division. *Americans with Disabilities Act Statutory Deadlines*. Washington, DC: GPO, 1990.

U.S. Preventive Services Task Force. *Guide to Clinical Preventive Services*. Baltimore: Williams & Wilkins, 1989.

Vernick, D. M. "What Did You Say? The Problem of Hearing Loss." *Brigham and Women's Hospital Medical Update* 2, no. 4 (November 1989): 1–5.

Vestibular Disorders Association. *Vestibular Disorders: What Are They?* Portland, OR: 1991.

Vestibular Disorders Association. *Diagnostic Tests for Vestibular Problems*. Portland, OR, 1992.

Watson, M. A., and H. Sinclair. *Balancing Act for People with Dizziness and Balance Disorders.* Portland, OR: Vestibular Disorders Association, 1992.

Weindruch, R., S. P. Korper, and E. Hadley. "The Prevalence of Disequilibrium and Related Disorders in Older Persons." *Ear, Nose and Throat Journal* 68 (December 1989): 925–929.

Weiss, G. "New Hope for Deaf Children." *American Health*, November 1990.

Weiss, R. "Travel Can Be Sickening: Now Scientists Know Why." *The New York Times*, April 28, 1992.

Williams, P. S., and L. Jacobs-Condit. *Hearing Aids: What Are They?* Washington, DC: National Information Center on Deafness/American Speech-Language-Hearing Association, 1991.

Wolfsen, R. J., H. Silverstein, F. I. Marlowe, and E. W. Keels. "Vertigo." *Clinical Symposia* 38, no. 6 (1986).

INDEX